A Guid
Canine Orthopa

A Guide to
Canine Orthopaedic Surgery

H. R. DENNY

MA, VetMB, PhD, FRCVS
Department of
Veterinary Surgery
University of Bristol

SECOND EDITION

BLACKWELL SCIENTIFIC PUBLICATIONS

OXFORD LONDON EDINBURGH

BOSTON PALO ALTO MELBOURNE

First published 1980
Second edition 1985

Photoset by Enset (Photosetting)
Midsomer Norton, Bath, Avon

Printed and bound in Great Britain
at The Alden Press, Oxford

DISTRIBUTORS

USA
  Blackwell Mosby Book
  Distributors
  11830 Westline Industrial Drive
  St Louis, Missouri 63141

Canada
  Blackwell Mosby Book
  Distributors
  120 Melford Drive, Scarborough
  Ontario M1B 2X4

Australia
  Blackwell Scientific Book
  Distributors
  31 Advantage Road, Highett
  Victoria 3190

British Library
Cataloguing in Publication Data

Denny, H.R.
  A guide to canine orthopaedic
  surgery.—2nd ed.
  1. Dogs—Diseases 2. Veterinary
  orthopedics
  I. Title
  636.7'08973   SF991

  ISBN 0-632-01272-2

Contents

vi

Preface

The first edition of this book was published in 1980. The aims of the second edition remain the same. The book is intended to be a guide to canine orthopaedic surgery in which conditions are described on a regional basis, instruction is simple and is freely illustrated with line drawings. It is hoped that this format will allow for rapid reference, both for students and busy practitioners trying to keep pace with current trends in veterinary surgery. The format does not allow for in–depth discussion, however references are provided at the end of each chapter for further reading. The second edition has been expanded to include important advances in canine orthopaedics made during the past 3 years, together with sections on bone disease, neoplasia, bandaging, external fixation techniques and tendon surgery, which were omitted in the first edition.

I gratefully acknowledge the continuing help of my colleagues at Langford and in practice who have made this book possible. Thanks are due to Valerie Beswetherick and Carol Francis who typed the manuscript.

H.R. DENNY

Chapter 1
Fractures

A fracture may be defined as a disruption in the continuity of a bone. The majority of fractures are caused by direct injury in road accidents or falls, the fracture occurring at or near the point of impact. A fracture may also be caused by an indirect force transmitted through bone or muscle to a vulnerable area of bone which breaks in a predictable manner; for example, fractures of the tibial tuberosity, olecranon or lateral condyle of the humerus. An inco-ordinate movement or excessive muscle contraction can result in this type of fracture. Factors which predispose to a fracture include the shape and position of the bone; hence long relatively exposed bones such as the radius and ulna and the tibia are more prone to fracture than the short compact bones of the carpus or tarsus.

The mechanical strength of a bone may be reduced locally by bone tumour formation or, generally, by disease caused by dietary or hormonal imbalance so that even minor trauma causes a fracture; this is called a pathological fracture.

THE CLASSIFICATION OF FRACTURES

Fractures may be classified according to:
1   External wounds.
2   Extent of bone damage.
3   Anatomical location and direction of the fracture line.
4   Relative displacement of the bone fragments.
5   Stability.

External wounds

A closed or simple fracture is one in which the overlying skin remains intact (Fig. 1) whereas an open or compound fracture is one in which there is a communication between the fracture site and a skin wound (Fig. 2).

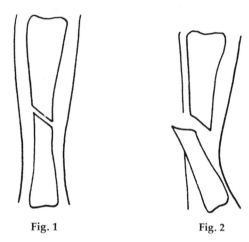

Fig. 1   Fig. 2

Extent of bone damage

A complete fracture is one in which there is total disruption in the continuity of the bone and usually marked displacement of the fragments.

An incomplete fracture is one in which partial continuity of the bone is maintained as in the green stick (bending) fractures of young animals (Fig. 3) or fissure fractures in adults (Fig. 4).

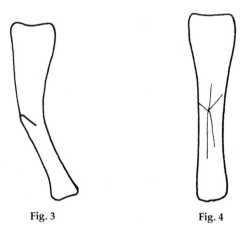

Fig. 3   Fig. 4

Anatomical location and direction of the fracture line

In classifying fractures by anatomical location, it is convenient to divide a typical long bone into 3 segments (Fig. 5).

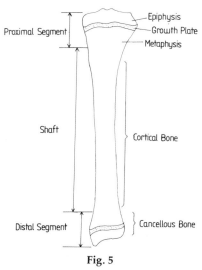

Fig. 5

1   The proximal epiphysis and the metaphysis consisting of cancellous bone.
2   The shaft consisting of cortical bone.
3   The distal metaphysis and epiphysis consisting of cancellous bone.
The fractures can then be described according to location — e.g. fracture of the proximal epiphysis or fracture of the shaft. Fractures of the epiphysis and growth plate injuries are divided into 6 types (Salter & Harris 1963) and these are described on page 68.
   Shaft fractures can be further classified according to the direction of the fracture line or the number of fragments.

Direction of fracture line

1   A transverse fracture is one in which the fracture line is at right angles to the long axis of the bone (Fig. 6).
2   An oblique fracture is one at an angle to the long axis of the bone (Fig. 7).

3

3   A spiral fracture curves around the bone (Fig. 8).
4   A comminuted fracture is one in which there are several fragments (Fig. 9).
5   A segmental fracture is one in which the bone is broken into three or more segments (Fig. 10).

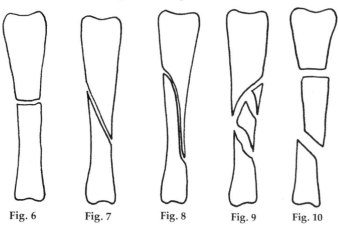

Fig. 6   Fig. 7   Fig. 8   Fig. 9   Fig. 10

Relative displacement of the fragments

1   A distraction or avulsion fracture is one in which a bone fragment is separated by the pull of the muscle, tendon or ligament which attaches to it, for example, fracture of the olecranon or avulsion of the tibial crest (Fig. 11).
2   An impacted fracture is one in which the fractured bone ends are driven into one another (Fig. 12).

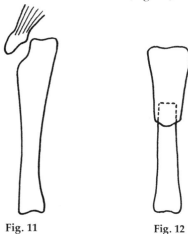

Fig. 11   Fig. 12

4

3 A compression fracture refers typically to fracture of a vertebra where a compressive force has resulted in shortening of a vertebra.

4 A depression fraction—this term is used to describe fractures of the skull in which the affected bone is 'pushed in', giving a concave deformity.

The stability of the fracture

A stable fracture is one in which the fragments interlock after reduction and resist shortening forces. The only fixation required in such a fracture is to prevent angular deformity. Most transverse fractures are in this category.

An unstable fracture is oblique or comminuted; here the fragments do not interlock following reduction and there is no resistance to shortening. Fixation is needed to maintain length, alignment and prevent rotation.

FRACTURE HEALING

The use of radiographs in the assessment of fracture healing

Radiography is essential to supplement clinical assessment of fracture healing and the following routine examination is used:

A.P. (Fig. 13) and lateral (Fig. 14) views are taken preoperatively.

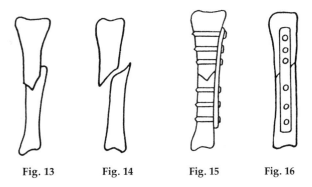

Fig. 13   Fig. 14   Fig. 15   Fig. 16

5

A.P. (Fig. 15) and lateral (Fig. 16) are taken post-operatively. When closed reduction is performed at least 50% of the fracture surfaces should be in contact if satisfactory healing is to occur (Fig. 17).

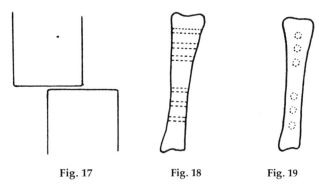

| Fig. 17 | Fig. 18 | Fig. 19 |

A.P. and lateral views are taken at 1 month.
A.P. and lateral views are taken at 2 months.
A.P. and lateral views are taken at 4 months when fracture healing is usually complete and implants can be removed as necessary (Figs 18 and 19).

Normal fracture healing

The radiographic features of fracture healing are easy to follow, provided the normal sequence of events which occurs during healing is understood.

A fracture is primarily bridged by two advancing collars of cartilage and woven bone (callus) which arise from the osteogenic layers of the periosteum and the endosteum (Figs 22, 23) Ham & Harris 1956). In an unstable fracture the callus consists mainly of cartilage but in a stable fracture woven or immature bone predominates. The cartilage or woven bone is next invaded by capillaries headed by osteo-clasts. At the same time osteoblasts lay down osteoid which matures to form bone, and collagen bundles are laid down in orderly lamellar fashion. In this way the initial scaffold of cartilage and woven bone which has stabilized the fracture is gradually replaced by mature lamellar bone. Remodelling by osteoclastic and osteoblastic activity is continued until the original shape of the bone is closely assumed again (Fig.

6

24). The final shape of the bone will conform to Wolff's law, i.e. 'that the internal architecture and external form of a bone are related to its function and change when the function is altered.'

Primary bone union

It is generally accepted that the function of callus is to stabilize the fragments and allow lamellar bone to grow and fill the fracture gap (Putnam & Pennock 1969); consequently, the size of the callus is related to the stability of the fracture (Hutzschemreuter *et al* 1969), and usually the more unstable the fracture the greater the size of the callus. A completely stable fracture should therefore heal without callus formation; this situation was investigated experimentally by Muller (1963). He made a hole in a pig's radius and found that healing took place without the participation of either the periosteum or the endosteum, the defect being filled by direct ingrowth of cortical bone. This type of healing was called primary bone union.

Rigid immobilization of a fracture can be achieved by internal fixation and compression of the fracture site. The aim of compression treatment of fractures is to achieve primary bone union in which direct longitudinal reconstruction of the bone occurs without any radiologically visible periosteal or endosteal callus (Muller *et al* 1970).

The rate of fracture healing

The rate of fracture healing is influenced by many factors.

AGE

The healing of fractures is more rapid in young animals; for example, in an immature dog union and remodelling of the fracture may be complete within 6 weeks, whereas in the mature dog it may be 4 months before remodelling is complete.

SPECIES OF ANIMAL

Clinically the rate of healing appears to vary with the

7

species so that healing appears to be slower in horses and cattle than in cats and dogs, but this may well be due to the mechanical factors involved in that it is far easier to immobilize fractures in small animals than in large.

TYPE OF BONE INVOLVED

Cancellous bone has an abundant blood supply and heals more rapidly than compact bone. Consequently fractures involving metaphysis or the epiphysis of a bone heal faster than those of the diaphysis.

THE TYPE OF FRACTURE

Impacted fractures and long spiral or oblique fractures where the fracture surfaces are in close relation heal faster than those in which there is wide distraction of the fragments. Comminuted fractures, where there are multiple fragments, tend to heal more slowly because of inherent instability and disruption of blood supply to the fragments. Fracture healing is also delayed by the presence of infection.

Radiographic changes during fracture healing
(Morgan 1972)

After reduction (Fig. 20) the first radiographic change at the fracture site occurs at 10 to 14 days when the fracture line becomes more distinct as a result of bone absorption along the fracture edges (Fig. 21).

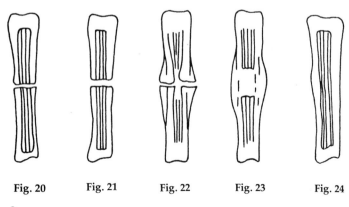

Fig. 20   Fig. 21   Fig. 22   Fig. 23   Fig. 24

8

The initial callus is uncalcified and is therefore not visible radiographically. The first reliable radiographic evidence that bone healing has commenced is the appearance of calcified periosteal callus (Fig. 22). Although the periosteal callus tends to obscure the endosteal callus, radiographically the endosteal callus contributes greatly to the disappearance of the fracture line (Fig. 23).

The late radiographic signs of bony union are: the restoration of the normal trabecular pattern which obscures the original fracture line, and remodelling and restoration of the continuity of the medullary cavity and cortex (Fig. 24).

These radiographic changes should be used to supplement clinical evidence of fracture union which may be briefly summarized as follows:

1   No pain on manipulation.
2   Stable fracture site.
3   Callus may be palpable depending on the method of fracture fixation.

COMPLICATIONS OF FRACTURE HEALING

The common complications of fracture healing include 'fracture disease', delayed and non–union, malunion, growth disturbances and osteomyelitis. 'Fracture disease' is a term used by Muller (1963) to describe the syndrome of muscle wasting, joint stiffness and osteoporosis, which results from prolonged immobilization of a limb during the healing of a fracture. One of the important advantages of rigid internal fixation of a fracture is that early pain free mobilization is possible and 'fracture disease' is avoided.

Delayed union and non–union

A frequent complication of fracture healing is delayed union. This is said to occur when a fracture has not healed in the time normally expected for that type of fracture. Delayed union may be superseded by the state of non–union, in which fracture healing stops and union will not

9

occur without surgical intervention. The clinical signs of non–union include painful motion at the fracture site, progressive deformity, disuse of the limb and muscle atrophy. The causes of delayed and non–union are the same and are listed below.

1 Inadequate immobilization.
2 Gap between fragments due to:
   (a) Soft tissue interposition.
   (b) Malalignment of the fragments.
   (c) Distraction of the fragments by traction or the improper use of internal fixation devices.
3 Loss of blood supply by:
   (a) Damage to the nutrient vessels of the bone.
   (b) Excessive stripping or injury to the periosteum.
   (c) Severe comminution.
4 Infection.
5 General factors which delay wound healing.

The commonest cause of delayed union or non–union is inadequate immobilization of the fracture. Fracture healing will proceed in the presence of a certain amount of tension, a considerable amount of bending will also be tolerated but torsion or rotation impedes healing because it results in tearing of the fibroblastic network of the callus. The prime objective in the treatment of non–unions is to provide adequate fixation but this presupposes that bone is capable of a biological response. Accordingly, Weber and Cech (1976) have classified non–union fractures into two broad groups.

1 Biologically active or viable non–unions.
2 Biologically inactive or non–viable non–unions.

The biologically active group includes 3 types of non–union:

i. *The hypertrophic type* is the commonest. This is seen as a complication of intramedullary pinning of humeral and femoral shaft fractures and is caused by rotation at the fracture site. Characteristically, a well vascularized 'elephant–shaped' foot callus develops which does not bridge the fracture gap. The gap contains cartilage and fibrous tissue. There is sclerosis of the bone ends and later the medullary cavity becomes sealed (Fig. 25a).

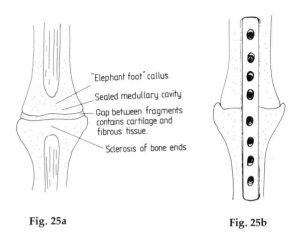

"Elephant foot" callus
Sealed medullary cavity
Gap between fragments contains cartilage and fibrous tissue.
Sclerosis of bone ends

Fig. 25a   Fig. 25b

When this type of non-union is rigidly immobilized, preferably with a compression plate, then the cartilage and fibrous tissue in the gap between the bone ends rapidly ossifies (Fig. 25b). Therefore, unless there is malalignment of the fracture, it is not necessary to 'freshen up' the bone ends (see atrophic non-union, p. 12) or to use a bone graft to stimulate osteogenesis. An intramedullary pin, if still present, must of course be removed before application of a plate.

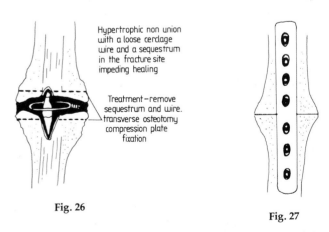

Hypertrophic non union with a loose cerclage wire and a sequestrum in the fracture site impeding healing

Treatment—remove sequestrum and wire. transverse osteotomy compression plate fixation

Fig. 26

Fig. 27

Other factors contributing to development of hyper-trophic non–union are loose cerclage wire and/or sequestrae (necrotic bone fragments) at the fracture site (Fig. 26). The fracture must be opened to remove these, necrotic bone is quite distinct from normal bone, it is yellowish–white in appearance and the margins of the fragment tend to have a 'chewed out' appearance. Following the debridement of the fracture site, if the bone ends are uneven, it is generally worth cutting back the bone 2–3 mm with a saw to give two flat surfaces which can be apposed and compressed with a plate (Fig. 27). This gives optimal stability and the best chance for union to occur.

ii. *Slightly hypertrophic type.* Instability following plate fixation may lead to this type of non–union in which there is minimal callus formation.

iii. *Oligotrophic type.* There is no callus formation and the fragments are usually widely separated and joined by fibrous tissue only. Failure to treat an avulsion fracture by internal fixation generally leads to an oligotrophic non–union.

All three types of biologically active non–union will usually heal provided rigid internal fixation is provided. The next group of non–unions, the biologically inactive or non–viable non–unions are not so easy to deal with. There are four types:

1 *The dystrophic type* is seen as a complication of comminuted fractures where a poorly revascularized fragment or fragments impedes fracture healing.

2 *The necrotic type* is also seen in comminuted or infected fractures where non–viable fragments or sequestrae at the fracture site impede healing.

3 *The defect type.* Here a major defect in the bone caused by removal of fragments or sequestrae is too big to be bridged by the normal healing process.

4 *The atrophic type.* This is the commonest and most difficult type of non–union to deal with. It is seen as a complication of fractures of the radius and ulna in Toy Poodles and miniature breeds of dog. There is instability at the fracture site with loss of osteogenic activity, osteoporosis and eventually osteolysis (Fig. 28). Shearing forces at the fracture site (Sumner–Smith & Cawley 1970) are thought to predispose to the non–union of the radius and ulna and

12

these occur if inadequate immobilization is achieved with a plaster cast. (Unless the cast is tight–fitting and extends from the foot to above the elbow, the dog is still able to rotate the upper forearm in the cast, causing shearing forces at the fracture site.) It is recommended that fresh fractures of the radius and ulna in toy and miniature breeds are treated by plate fixation whenever possible to avoid non–union and the ASIF mini–compression plates (Straumann Great Britain Ltd) are ideal for this purpose.

The prime objective in treating avascular non–unions is to stimulate osteogenesis. The fracture site is exposed, cartilage and fibrous tissue are excised and the bone ends are 'freshened up' by cutting back the bone 1–2 mm (Fig. 29). The fracture is stabilized with a plate and a cancellous bone graft is taken from the proximal humerus and packed around the fracture site to stimulate osteogenesis. If despite these measures, non–union of the radius and ulna persists, then repeat operations are rarely successful in giving union and amputation should be considered.

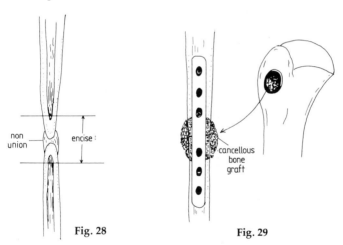

Fig. 28   Fig. 29

Malunion

Malunion is defined as a fracture that has healed or is healing in an abnormal position. Causes are improper reduction and/or immobilization during in healing.

13

Growth disturbance

Trauma to a growth plate with or without fracture may cause premature closure and result in shortening of the limb or angular deformity.

Compound fractures and osteomyelitis

Normal periosteum provides bone with an adequate defence against invading organisms, but when this protection is removed as a result of a fracture or surgery then the bone becomes extremely susceptible to infection (Peacock & Van Winkle 1970). The *ideal* treatment of compound fractures should therefore be aimed at restoring the continuity of the periosteum and protecting it so that it may in turn defend the bone against infection; this can be achieved by perfect open reduction, rigid internal fixation, debridement and wide excision of the wound, followed by primary closure of the soft tissue.

Primary bacterial contamination occurs in only about a third of compound fractures; any necrotic tissue which is left in the wound serves as a nidus for bacterial multiplication. Secondary bacterial infection of the wound occurs after six to eight hours (Muller *et al* 1970). Although the ideal method of treatment of compound fractures has been mentioned, there are risks, especially when metal implants are used in a potentially infected bone and so the cautious surgeon will vary the ideal method as necessary.

When the compound fracture is less than 8 hours old, there is minimal soft tissue damage and no gross contamination of the wound with foreign material then the wound may be safely excised and sutured. The fracture can be treated by internal fixation or external fixation at this stage depending on its location and type. If internal fixation is used the reduction of the fracture is best made through a clean surgical incision at some distance from the wound.

When a compound fracture is over 8 hours old or there is gross contamination or soft tissue damage; then, following a thorough debridement and excision, the wound is left open and covered with a protective bandage. External

14

fixation, or a Kirschner splint (see p. 42), is used to stabilize the fracture until union is complete, or internal fixation is subsequently carried out between one and three weeks provided that the original wound is healing with no evidence of infection. Open reduction and internal fixation is again carried out through a fresh surgical incision through healthy tissue. Primary internal fixation may be occasionally necessary in this second category of compound fractures; if so, installation of a drainage tube is useful as it will allow continual drainage and also direct irrigation of the fracture site with the appropriate antibiotic solution. Irrigation drainage is maintained for a week post-operatively. Whatever method is used, parenteral antibiotic cover should be given for at least three weeks.

Osteomyelitis does however occur as a complication of compound fractures and puncture wounds (Hickman 1967), and also unfortunately as one of the most common complications following the surgical treatment of fractures (Vaughan 1975). Organisms most frequently isolated from the infected bone in dogs include species of staphylococcus, streptococcus, pasteurella, pseudomonas, proteus and coliforms (Vaughan 1975).

Haematogenous spread of infection is rare; it may be seen in young animals when infection localizes in a damaged area of bone (usually the metaphysis) during the course of a bacteraemia.

When the focus of infection is within the medullary cavity there is rapid spread throughout it, pus penetrates the cortex, underruns the periosteum, breaks out and escapes through sinuses in the skin. Areas of cortical bone may lose their blood supply and become necrotic. The necrotic area of bone gradually separates as a sequestrum and becomes walled off by fibrous tissue and an area of dense new bone which is called an involucrum. Infection of the medullary cavity is known as osteomyelitis whereas localized infection of the periosteum or cortical bone are respectively known as periostitis and osteitis.

The clinical signs of osteomyelitis include soft tissue swelling, pain, sinus formation and intermittent pyrexia. Radiographic examination reveals areas of rarefaction in the bone, particularly in the metaphyses or around the metal implants such as pins, screws or plates which may have been used to stabilize a fracture (Fig. 30). Later there is periosteal new bone formation and if a sequestrum develops this will appear as an area of increased density in the bone surrounded by a zone of decreased density or osteolysis (Fig. 31).

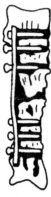

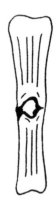

Fig. 30   Fig. 31

Low grade infection may be controlled by the administration of the appropriate antibiotic as determined by culture and sensitivity examination. Therapy should be continued for at least three weeks. In established cases of osteomyelitis adequate drainage must be provided and all sequestrae, necrotic bone and where necessary, metallic implants removed. Irrigation drainage is usually maintained for a week post-operatively.

Although infection delays healing of fractures union will occur provided the fracture is stable (Muller *et al* 1970). Fractures complicated by osteomyelitis and non−union are best treated by thorough debridement of the infected bone followed by rigid immobilization of the fracture preferably with a plate (Vaughan 1975). Where there is active infection treatment can be carried out in two stages, firstly sequestrae and implants are removed and the appropriate antibiotic given for 7 to 10 days. At the second operation debridement is completed and the fracture stabilized with a plate. Large defects in the bone may be filled with a graft of chips of

16

autogenous cancellous bone. Irrigation drainage of the fracture site is advisable in conjunction with a prolonged course of antibiotic therapy.

Bone grafts

Bone grafts are used to promote healing of non-union fractures, to fill defects in bone resulting from fractures, osteomyelitis, cysts or tumours, and for the arthrodesis (fusion) of joints. Bone grafts heal by a process of 'creeping substitution' (Ham & Leeson 1961). Most of the transplanted cells die and are gradually replaced by mesenchymal cells from the host bed which differentiate to form osteoblasts and osteoclasts. This process occurs more rapidly within the relatively porous structure of cancellous bone.

It is generally agreed that the healing process is most rapid when autogenous grafts are used, but although there is a delay in the healing rate of homogenous grafts this is not significant enough to affect their use clinically (Vaughan 1972). Heterogenous bone, however, is far less readily incorporated into the host site.

Bone grafts serve three main functions, they provide a scaffold in which new bone can be laid down, they provide a local source of calcium and minerals, and cause increased osteogenesis because of their nature or by osseous metaplasia of the surrounding connective tissue.

There is considerable clinical and some experimental evidence that fresh autogenous cancellous bone grafts promote fracture healing, and this is probably due to the inductive properties of the matrix of the graft rather than the provision of cells with osteoblastic activity (Peacock & Van Winkle 1970). Cancellous bone grafts also 'survive well' in the presence of infection and are useful to promote healing of fractures complicated by osteomyelitis. Suitable sites for collection of an autogenous cancellous bone graft include the proximal humerus, femur and tibia. An osteotome or trephine is used to make a window in the cortical bone through which a curette is introduced and used to scrape out the cancellous bone. Another common site of collection is the wing of the ilium. The cancellous bone graft should be collected in a dry, sterile glass container and transferred to the recipient site as quickly as possible. The graft is packed in and around the site and held in place by carefully suturing the surrounding soft tissues. Cortical bone grafts possess rigidity and strength and can be used like a bone plate to restore the continuity of a bone. This type of graft acts purely as a scaffold and is gradually replaced by bone from the recipient site. Rigid immobilization of the graft is essential during this healing process. Cortical grafts seldom survive in the presence of infection and are rejected as sequestra. A source of fresh autogenous cortical bone is the rib but homogenous cortical bone grafts are equally satisfactory. The advantage of using a homogenous bone graft is that it avoids the necessity of two operations on the same animal and also it can be stored in a variety of shapes and sizes ready for use. Homogenous bone grafts can be collected from a donor animal immediately after euthanasia provided the bone is collected with strictly aseptic precautions. These grafts may then be stored in sterile containers at $-20°C$ and used at any time up to six months after collection.

Nutritional disorders of bone (Bennett 1976)

An adequate dietary intake of calcium, phosphorus and Vitamin D is needed for the development and maintenance of normal bone. The requirements for dogs have been estimated (Krook 1971) as:

1 Calcium 265 mg/kg bodyweight/day
2 Phosphorus 220 mg/kg bodyweight/day
3 Vitamin D 7 iu/kg bodyweight/day

These figures apply to adult dogs; puppies need twice this intake. It is important to feed the correct ratio of calcium to phosphorus otherwise a relative deficiency of one or other occurs. The calcium to phosphorus ratio should be 1:1. In most diets there tends to be an excess of phosphorus—for example in meat the ratio of phosphorus to calcium is 20:1. A diet of meat and water rapidly leads to calcium deficiency but carnivores in the wild avoid this problem by eating the bones of their victims which are a natural balanced source of calcium and phosphorus. The growing puppy will need about 50% of meat in the diet initially which is gradually reduced to 30–40%—the rest is made up with carbohydrate and vegetable. If the puppy is receiving a balanced diet, the natural way of supplementing calcium and phosphorus is to give milk and bone meal. The latter is given at a rate of 15–20 grams/kg dry weight of food (Abrams 1962). It should be stressed however, that bone meal will not correct an abnormal dietary calcium/phosphorus ratio. If the puppy is calcium deficient, then calcium lactate is given (available in 300 mg tablets—Evans).

Vitamin D is needed for the absorption of calcium from the bowel. Natural sources of the vitamin are meat, milk, eggs and sunlight. Supplements are given as necessary as cod liver oil capsules (5 ml cod liver oil/10 kg bodyweight for daily growth).

Nutritional secondary hyperparathyroidism
('All Meat Syndrome'. Juvenile osteoporosis, osteogenesis imperfecta)

Nutritional secondary hyperparathyroidism results from calcium deficiency, either due to lack of dietary calcium or a relative deficiency due to excess dietary phosphorus. The condition is seen most frequently in dogs fed on all meat diets, in which calcium levels are low and phosphorus are high. Other causes are: inability to absorb or utilize dietary calcium (true osteogenesis imperfecta) which is seen in some lines of Alsatian puppies, or reduced availability of dietary calcium as in Vitamin D deficiency or renal insufficiency.

Calcium deficiency causes hypocalcaemia and parathyroid hormone release. Calcium is resorbed from the skeleton to maintain normal blood calcium levels (9–12 mg/ 100 ml serum). Clinical features of the condition include lameness, pain, difficulty in standing, bone deformity and pathological fractures. The fractures tend to involve the spine and hind limbs. Radiographic examination reveals generalized loss of bone density, thin cortices and pathological fractures.

Treatment

Obviously the meat rich diet should be terminated and substituted with a nutritionally balanced diet supplemented with calcium lactate. Analgesics are given as necessary to control pain. Vitamin D supplementation should be avoided, especially in the early stages of treatment because it promotes further bone absorption and may aggravate the condition. Severely affected puppies, particularly those which are paraplegic or those with several pathological fractures, should be destroyed on humane grounds.

Hypertrophic osteodystrophy (Skeletal scurvy, Barlow's disease)

Hypertrophic osteodystrophy is seen in the larger breeds of dog between four and six months of age. The aetiology of the condition is uncertain but it tends to be seen in rapidly growing puppies that are having excessive vitamin and mineral supplements. Vitamin C deficiency has also been suggested as a cause but although vitamin C has proved useful in treatment it should be realized that dogs are capable of synthesizing their own vitamin C.

Clinical signs

The metaphyses of the longbones, especially the distal radius and distal tibia, become enlarged, warm and painful. Affected animals are reluctant to move and an intermittent high fever is often noted. The radiographic changes associated with hypertrophic osteodystrophy are summarized in Fig. 31a.

Most animals recover in one two two months provided strict rest is given, the excess vitamin and mineral supplements are curtailed and a light diet is given. Campbell (1964) has found the administration of vitamin C (oral dose 0.5–1 gram per day) useful in the treatment. Analgesics and anti–inflammatory drugs are used to relieve pain and pyrexia. Although dogs may have a complete remission of clinical signs, relapses do occasionally occur during the remaining growth period.

20

Rickets (Campbell 1964)

Rickets is a name which is often loosely and wrongly used to describe nutritional bone disorders in young dogs. Clinically, the disease is now very rare. It probably results from a dietary deficiency of vitamin D, calcium and/or phosphorus. Vitamin D deficiency results in a cartilage matrix that is highly stable and does not calcify. In young animals this results in thickened and irregular growth plates, mushrooming of the metaphyses, softening and bending of bones.

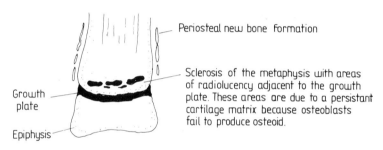

Periosteal new bone formation

Sclerosis of the metaphysis with areas of radiolucency adjacent to the growth plate. These areas are due to a persistant cartilage matrix because osteoblasts fail to produce osteoid.

Growth plate

Epiphysis

Fig. 31a

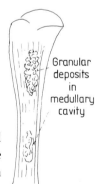

Granular deposits in medullary cavity

Fig. 31b

Eosinophilic panosteitis (Bohning et al 1970)

Although panosteitis is commonly seen in the United States, it is rare in this country (Tandy 1977). It affects the longbones of large breeds of dog especially the German Shepherd. Lameness is sudden in onset, it may last a few days or several weeks and tends to shift from leg to leg. The recurring bouts of lameness usually subside by the time the dog reaches two years of age. There is pain on palpation of affected bones and, on X–ray, granular deposits or sclerotic areas are seen in the medullary cavity (Fig. 31b). Treatment is symptomatic, analgesics or corticosteroids being given to relieve pain.

21

Hypertrophic pulmonary osteopathy (HPOA. Alexander *et al* 1965)

Hypertrophic pulmonary osteopathy is seen as a complication of chronic pulmonary disease and results in periosteal proliferation. It is most frequently associated with pulmonary neoplasia. The distal parts of the limb become swollen and painful and there is obvious lameness. The classical radiographic signs consist of extensive, rough periosteal new bone formation beginning on the distal phalanges, metacrpal bones and metatarsal bones. Other bones may become involved. If the primary lesion in the lung can be removed, regression of symptoms will occur. Generally, however, treatment is not feasible.

Craniomandibular osteopathy (Riser, Parkes and Shirer 1967)

This condition is seen particularly in West Highland Terriers and has led to the name 'Westie's Disease'. Other Terrier breeds are also susceptible. The cause is not known but the lesion is essentially a periostitis with new bone formation on the ventral borders of the horizontal mandibular rami and around the tympanic bullae. There is obvious swelling of the jaws, inappetence, lethargy and pyrexia. Symptoms become apparent between three and six months of age. Puppies will show pain on palpation of the mandible or on opening the jaws. The condition tends to run an undulant course and regress at about one year of age. Corticosteroids generally provide effective relief from symptoms.

Bone tumours

Bone tumours in the dog can be classified as follows:

Benign bone tumours
Osteoma.
Osteochondroma.
Enchondroma.

22

Benign Chondroblastoma.
Osteoclastoma.
Bone cyst.
Non–ossyfing fibroma.

Malignant bone tumours
Osteosarcoma.
Chondrosarcoma.
Fibrosarcoma.
Malignant Giant Cell Tumour.

Allied malignant lesions of bone
Reticulum Cell Sarcoma.
Multiple Myeloma.
Haemangiosarcoma.
Haemopericytoma.

Metastatic bone tumours

It is important for the orthopaedic surgeon to be able to differentiate between benign and malignant bone tumours. Unfortunately the majority of bone tumours encountered in the dog are malignant and the osteosarcoma accounts for 80% of tumours of the skeletal system. Benign bone tumours and also metastatic bone tumours are uncommon in animals. Osteosarcoma are found in the large and giant breeds of dog and it is generally the older animal that is affected but cases have been recorded in dogs as young as one year of age. The primary tumour is usually found in the metaphyseal region of a longbone and the predeliction sites are the proximal humerus, the distal radius, the distal femur

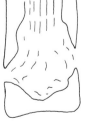

Destruction of cortical bone

Growth of the tumour beyond the original confines of the bone

Fig. 31c

Fig. 31d

23

and the proximal tibia, but any part of the skeleton can be affected. The tumour presents as a hard, often painful swelling. The radiographic changes associated with osteosarcomas have been described by Morgan 1972 (see Figs 31c,d,e). These include destruction of cortical bone, growth of the tumour beyond the original confines of the bone and development of a tumour mass that may become ossified or may contain calcified material. Osteosarcomas appear radiographically to be one of three types:

(a) osteoblastic
(b) Osteoclastic, which is slightly more common, and
(c) a mixture of osteoblastic and osteoclastic.

Approximately 50% of osteosarcomas give rise to a 'sunburst' effect which is a reaction of the periosteum to produce radiating spicules of new bone.

Osteosarcomas seldom invade joint spaces or adjacent bones. However, changes due to pressure deformity and periosteal reaction may be seen on radiographs. Osteosarcomas rarely follow trauma and it is probably coincidental that a tumour develops at an old fracture site.

Early radiographic diagnosis of osteosarcoma is not always easy. If there is any doubt about the radiographic diagnosis then the examination should be repeated approximately four weeks later when typical changes associated with the tumour should have become apparent.

The prognosis is generally hopeless because osteosarcomas are highly malignant and metastasize to the lungs. Chest radiographs should be taken, however very few cases have radiographic evidence of lung metastases when the primary tumour is identified. Euthanasia should be recommended on diagnosis and treatment by amputation is seldom justified because affected animals have to be destroyed within six months of surgery because of lung metastases.

Bone cysts

Bone cysts are occasionally encountered in the dog and the literature on these lesions has been reviewed by Carrig, Pool & McElroy (1975). The cyst is generally found in the metaphyseal region of either the distal radius or ulna, femur or tibia. Young dogs of the large breeds are affected, a painless bony swelling develops and radiographs show a radiolucent lesion with marked thinning of the overlying cortices (Fig. 31f). There is no evidence of an actively destructive process or of any reactive periosteal new bone present. Trabeculation within the cysts is minimal. The cyst should be drained, the cavity curetted and then packed with a cancellous bone graft. The response to surgery is usually good and the cyst decreases in size while the bone cortices thicken.

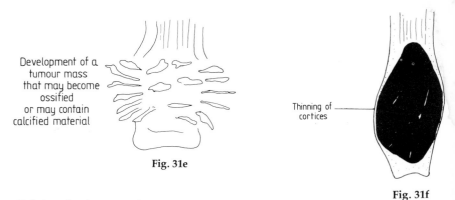

Development of a tumour mass that may become ossified or may contain calcified material

Fig. 31e

Thinning of cortices

Fig. 31f

Calcinosis circumscripta

Calcinosis circumscripta is the name given to a granulo-matous lesion which consists of chalky/putty–like masses embedded in fibrous tissue. The condition is seen most often in the German Shepherd and affected animals are under one year of age. Lesions may be single or multiple and can be found in a variety of sites, such as the foot, closely attached to the cervical vertebrae, the thorax, elbow, ischium and even under the tongue. The lesions are benign and they can be excised. However, surgical excision may be difficult because of the firm soft tissue attachments. Cal-cinosis circumscripta lesions in the neck are closely attached to the cervical vertebrae and excision carries a real risk of damage to the nerve roots to the brachial plexus. In this site, therefore, surgical treatment should be avoided. There is a tendency for the lesion to stop growing and, in fact, to regress by the time the dog reaches one year of age. The aetiology of calcinosis circumscripta is unknown but it has

25

been described as an inherited local metabolic defect of connective tissue (Seawright & Grono, 1961).

JOINT INJURY

A diarthrodial joint (Fig. 32) consists essentially of two opposing bone surfaces which are covered with hyaline cartilage and joined peripherally by a joint capsule. The articular surface of the bone is composed of compact bone covered with hyaline cartilage. The cartilage has no nerve or blood supply and it is generally accepted that it derives its nutrition from synovial fluid. The cartilage is well adapted to counter concussion and friction by means of its structure and lubrication by synovial fluid. Although microscopically chrondrocytes show no sign of activity, it has been demonstrated that the turnover of the matrix is rapid, indeed far greater than could possibly be required to replenish wear and tear over areas of high pressure (Mankin & Lippiello 1969). The matrix which is continuously produced by chrondrocytes is broken down at the same time by proteolytic enzymes in particular cathepsin D (Bassett 1966). This process of autolysis occurs in the substance of cartilage rather than on the surface and normally the balance between anabolism and catabolism is so precise that the thickness of the matrix varies little throughout life.

Repair of articular cartilage depends on the depth and position of the defect. Superficial defects in the cartilage never heal unless they are close to the attachment of the synovial membrane, whereas a wound which extends through cartilage to the sub-chrondal bone is gradually filled with fibrocartilage (Meacham & Roberts 1971), Vaughan & Robins 1975). Joint instability results in fibrous tissue hypertrophy. This tissue is replaced by plaques of cartilage which later undergo endochrondral ossification to form osteophytes. These changes occur particularly at the transitional zone of the joint which is the junction between periosteum, synovial membrane and articular cartilage. The area has a profuse blood supply.

The joint capsule consists of two layers (Fig. 32), the outer

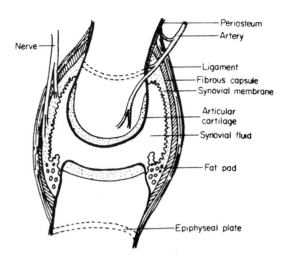

Nerve

Periosteum
Artery
Ligament
Fibrous capsule
Synovial membrane
Articular cartilage
Synovial fluid
Fat pad
Epiphyseal plate

Fig. 32

fibrous layer which is thickened in parts to form ligaments and the inner layer or synovial membrane which is responsible for the secretion and absorption of synovial fluid. The synovial membrane has a rich supply of arteries, lymphatics and nerves, its surfaces are covered with fine villi which hypertrophy in disease.

The component structures of a joint may be torn or stretched when a joint is forced beyond its normal range of physiological movement, in a fall or inco-ordinate movement; alternatively injury may be precipitated by the abnormal structure and hence abnormal movement of the joint as in hip dysplasia, or by excessive wear and tear in the old or overweight animal. Whatever the initial cause a sequence of events follows which is called osteo-arthrosis or Degenerative Joint Disease (Sten-Erik Olsson 1971).

Injury to areas of articular cartilage results in loss of elasticity, softening and later fissure formation. Chrondroitin sulphate is released from the damaged cartilage and this provokes an inflammatory response at the synovial membrane. Grossly the membrane becomes thickened and secretes increased amounts of synovial fluid. At the same time the fibrous joint capsule undergoes a normal inflammatory response with increased vascularity and swelling. Later there is fibrous thickening of the capsule and the development of osteophytes, particularly at the transitional zone of the joint.

The tissue changes, especially degeneration of the articular cartilage, are irreversible and treatment should be aimed at preventing the progression of the disease as soon as possible. This may be achieved by rest for at least a month. The administration of analgesics and anti-inflammatory drugs, such as corticosteroids, can be useful to control the pain associated with the disease but only when strict rest is enforced, otherwise premature use of the joint may result in further damage.

Corticosteroids remain one of the most effective groups of agent used for the relief of symptoms of joint disease because they inhibit all stages of inflammation. Short term administration is usually well tolerated but the longterm systemic use of corticosteroids is associated with undesirable side effects. Repeated intra–articular corticosteroid injections may lead to cartilage destruction (Mankin 1974).

Conditions that are particularly amenable to corticosteroid therapy include acute non–traumatic arthritis, osteoarthritis uncomplicated by joint deformity and traumatic arthritis without fracture of the articular cartilage or derangement of the joint. Corticosteroids are not so effective in the treatment of chronic osteoarthritis associated with extensive periarticular osteophyte formation.

Non–steroidal anti–inflammatory drugs are preferred for the treatment of chronic osteoarthritis. They can be divided into 5 groups (Short & Beadle 1978) which are listed below:

A. Salicylates
1   Acetoxy–5–acetylsalicylic acid.
2   Aspirin—25 mg/kg divided into 2 daily doses is usually well tolerated.
3   Salicylamide.
4   Sodium salicylate.

B. Pyrazolon Derivatives
1   Acetaminophen (paracetamol).
2   Aminopyrine.

28

3   Antipyrine.
4   Oxyphenbutazone.
5   Phenylbutazone—For chronic use 1–2 mg/kg divided into 2 or 3 daily doses. Higher dose rates for acute flare ups of joint pain—4–5 mg/kg divided into 2 or 3 daily doses. Longterm side effects—bone marrow suppression.
6   Sulfinpyrazone.

C. Fenamic Acid Derivatives
1   Flufenamic acid.
2   Meclofenamic acid.
3   Mefenamic acid—Ponstan (Parke Davis) 12 mg/kg divided into 2 daily doses given with food.

D. Indene and Related Derivatives
1   Benzydamine.
2   Fenamole.
3   Indomethacin—1–1.25 mg/kg divided into 2–3 daily doses. Serious gastrointestinal problems can occur with chronic use.
4   Indoxole.

F. Arylalkanoic Acids
1   Ibuprofen—15 mg/kg divided into 3 daily doses given with food.
2   Ketoprofen.
3   Naproxen.

Prednoleucotropin (Cinophen, Hexamine, Prednisolone, Sodium Salicylate) is another preparation (in which the anti–inflammatory activity of prednisolone is enhanced by other active ingredients) that has proved useful in the treatment of osteoarthritis.

Surgery may be needed to treat the original cause of the osteoarthritis, for example the repair of a ligament to restore joint stability, or later to remove osteophytes which may be interfering with joint function.

Infectious arthritis

Although haematogenous spread of infection to joints is

common in young farm animals, the condition is rare in the dog. Direct infection as a complication of a penetrating wound, arthrotomy, or by extension of infection from a local purulent focus occur more frequently. The sequence of pathological changes are similar to but far more marked than in osteo-arthrosis, with rapid and extensive destruction of areas of articular cartilage and subchondral bone. Later there is marked periarticular new bone formation which may eventually result in ankylosis of the joint.

Clinical examination reveals a hot, swollen, extremely painful joint and if the joint is open there will be a discharge of pus and synovial fluid. Treatment of infective arthritis involves removal of purulent material from the joint; this is done by aspiration through a needle in closed cases and by flushing the joint out with sterile normal saline in open cases. The joint is irrigated with aqueous penicillin or other appropriate antibiotic solution. Open cases are protected with a bandage and left to heal by granulation. Prolonged parenteral antibiotic therapy is essential. In chronic cases surgical debridement and synoviectomy may be necessary to eradicate the infection. Even when infection has been eradicated pain may persist as a result of the extensive destruction of the joint surfaces, and this pain may only be relieved by arthrodesis of the joint or amputation of the limb.

Rheumatoid arthritis (Newton & Lipowitz 1975; Biery & Newton 1975)

Rheumatoid arthritis is comparatively rare in the dog. Immune complexes form in the joints and erosion of cartilage occurs causing severe and often progressive polyarthritis. The condition has been recorded most frequently in Shelties, Collies and Dachsunds. There is lameness, swelling and pain associated with several joints. The carpus and hock are most frequently affected. The American Rheumatism Association use 11 criteria, listed below, to establish a diagnosis of rheumatoid arthritis and at least 9 of these should be present to confirm the diagnosis in the dog.

1   Morning stiffness.

2   Pain or tenderness on joint motion.

3   Swelling of at least one joint (soft tissue or fluid).

4   Swelling of any other joint.

5   Symmetrical onset of joint swelling and symptoms.

6   Subcutaneous nodules.

7   Radiographic changes typical of RA.

8   Positive rheumatoid factor—by a reliable method.

9   Poor mucin precipitate of synovial fluid.

10   Characteristic histological synovial changes. Villous projection of the synovium with lymphoid and plasma cell infiltration.

11   Characteristic histological findings of nodules.

The classical radiographic changes associated with rheumatoid arthritis are flask shaped destructive lesions in the subchondral bone. Treatment can only be palliative and salicylates (Aspirin) provide the most effective relief.

Systemic lupus erythrematosus (Krum *et al* 1977)

Systemic lupus erythrematosus (SLE) is a complex disorder characterized by the development of one or all of the following clinical syndromes:

Haemolytic anaemia.

Thrombocytopaenic purpura.

Glomerulonephritis.

Polyarthritis.

SLE is an autoimmune disease and diagnosis is based on the demonstration of antinuclear antibodies. Polyarthritis due to SLE should be differentiated from rheumatoid arthritis—erosions in the articular cartilage are not seen so frequently as in the latter. Another feature of SLE is joint instability, caused by degenerative changes in the supporting ligaments, this is seen particularly in the carpus and the stifle. Dogs with SLE are treated with high doses of Prednisolone. The long term prognosis is poor.

THE HEALING OF TENDONS

Mature tendons consist essentially of tightly packed

bundles of collagen in which fibrocytes are interspersed. The blood supply is poor and is derived mainly from the mesotendon which is a synovial membrane lying between the tendon and its sheath. Tendons heal slowly but healing of the sheath is much more rapid. When a tendon is severed, the resultant wound is invaded by fibroblasts derived from the paratenon (Skoog & Persson 1954). They defined the paratenon as the subcutaneous connective tissue, i.e. the fascia, surrounding a tendon. The fibroblasts lay down randomly orientated collagen fibrils. The collagen fibrils then become organized so that by three months post-injury they are found to be longitudinally orientated between the severed tendon ends and randomly orientated in the surrounding tissues (Peacock 1964). Macroscopically the scar filling the gap is difficult to distinguish from normal tendinous tissue. Mason & Allen (1961) investigated the tensile strength of tendons during the healing process and found that function of the tendon during the early stages of exudation, fibroplasia and fibrous union had a deleterious effect on healing whereas function of the tendon during the stage of maturation and organization accelerated the process. Consequently, following tendon repair complete immobilization is essential for one month post-operatively and then a gradual increase in movement is allowed during the following two months. In tendon repair restoration of tensile strength is a prime objective, but at the same time gliding function should be maintained if normal limb movement is to continue. Gliding function of the tendon is commonly complicated by excessive scar tissue formation; this can be minimized by the surgical techniques employed in the repair and also by controlled exercise during the latter stages of healing.

THE HEALING OF MUSCLE

In general damaged muscle is replaced by scar tissue (Walter & Israel 1967). However, in voluntary striated muscle limited regeneration may occur so that although the continuity of a surgical incision is restored primarily by

fibrous tissue, this may later be replaced by muscle if sarco-
lemmal proliferation occurs.

REFERENCES

ALEXANDER J.E., KEOWN G.H. & PATOLAY J.L. (1963) Granular cell myo-
blastoma with hypertrophic osteopathy in a mare. *J. Am. Vet. Med.
Ass.* **146,** 703.

BASSETT C.A.C. (1966) *Cartilage Degradation and Repair.* Proceedings of a
Workshop, Washington D.C. National Academy of Sciences, National
Research Council.

BENNETT D. (1976) Nutrition and bone disease in the dog and cat. *Vet. Rec.*
98, 313.

BIERY D.N. & Newton C.D. (1975) Radiographic appearance of rheumatoid
arthritis in the dog. *J. Am. Anim. Hosp. Ass.* **11,** 607.

BOHNING R., SUTER P., HOHN R.B. & MARSHALL J. (1970) Clinical and radiological survey of canine panosteitis. *J. Am. Vet. Med. Ass.* 870–884.

CAMPBELL J.R. (1964) *J. small Anim. Pract.* **5,** 229.

CARRIG L.B., POOL R.R. and McELROY J.M. (1975) Polyostatic cystic bone
lesions in a dog. *J. small Anim. Pract.* **16,** 495.

HAM A.W. & HARRIS W.R. (1956) Repair and transplantation of bone; in:
The Biochemistry and Physiology of Bone. New York Ac. Ad. Press.

HAM A.W. & LEESON T.S. (1961) *Histology,* 4th edn. J.B. Lipincott Co,
Philadelphia and Montreal.

HICKMAN J. (1967) *Veterinary Orthopaedics.* Oliver & Boyd Ltd, London.

KRUM S.H., CARDINET G.H., ANDERSON B.C. & HOLLIDAY T.A. (1977) Poly-
moysitis and polyarthritis associated with systemic lupus erythrematosus in the dog. *J. Am. Vet. Med. Ass.* **170,** 61.

MANKIN H.J. & LIPPIELLO L. (1970) Biochemical and metabolic abnormalities
in articular cartilage from osteoarthritic human hips. *J. Bone Joint Surg.*
52A, 424.

MANKIN H.J. (1974) The reaction of articular cartilage to injury and osteoarthritis In: *Engl. J. Med.* **291,** 1285.

MASON M.L. & ALLEN H.C. (1961) Rate of healing in tendon–an experimental study of tensile strength. *Ann. Surg.* **113,** 424.

MEACHIM G. & ROBERTS C. (1971) Repair of the joint surface from sub-
articular tissue in the rabbit knee. *J. Anat.* **109,** 317.

MORGAN J.P. (1972) *Radiology in Veterinary Orthopedics.* p. 122. Lea &
Febiger, Philadelphia.

MULLER M.E. (1963) Internal fixation for fresh fractures and for non-union.
Proc. Roy. Soc. Med. **56,** 455.

MULLER M.E., ALLGOWER M. & WILLENEGER H. (1970) *Manual of Internal
Fixation.* Springer Verlag, Berlin, Heidelberg, New York.

NEWTON C.D. & LIPOWITZ A.J. (1975) Canine rheumatoid arthritis: a brief
review. *J. Am. Anim. Hosp. Ass.* **11,** 595–606.

OLSSON STEN-ERIK (1971) Degenerative joint disease (osteoarthrosis): a
review with special reference to the dog. *J. small Anim. Pract.* **12,** 333.

OWEN L.N. & WALKER R.C. (1963) Osteitis fibrosa cystica of the radius in an
Irish Wolfhound. *Vet. Rec.* **75,** 40.

33

PEACOCK E.A. (1964) Fundamental aspects of wound repair relating to the reconstruction of gliding function after tendon repair. *Surg. Gynec. & Obstet.* **119,** 241.

PEACOCK E.. & VAN WINKEL W. (1970) *The Surgery and Biology of Wound Repair.* W.B. Saunders & Co, Philadelphia, London & Toronto.

PUTNAM R.W. & PENNOCK E.W. (1969) Compression plating in veterinary orthopaedics. *Mod. Vet. Pract.* **00,** 28.

RISER W.F., PARKES L.J. & SHIRER J.F. (1967) Canine craniomandibular osteopathy. *J. Am. Vet. Radiol. Soc.* **8,** 23.

SALTER R.B. & HARRIS W.R. (1963) Injuries involving the epiphyseal plate. *J. Bone. Jt. Surgery.* **45A,** 587.

SEAWRIGHT A.A. and GRONO L.R. (1961) Calcinosis Circumscripta in Dogs. *Aust. Vet. J.* **37,** 421.

SHORT P.R. & BEADLE R.E. (1978) Pharmacology of anti–arthritic drugs. *Vet. Clinics of N. America,* Vol. **8,** 401.

SITTNIKOW K. & PAATSAMA S. (1970) The healing of distal fractures of the radius and ulna. *J. small Anim. Pract.* **11,** 305.

SKOOG T. & PERSSON B.H. (1954) An experimental study of early healing of tendons. *Plast. & Reconstruct Surg.* **13,** 384.

SUMNER-SMITH G. & CAWLEY A.J. (1970) Non–union of fractures in the dog. *J. small Anim. Pract.* **11,** 311–325.

TANDY J. (1977) A case of panosteitis. *Vet. Rec.* **100,** 287.

VAUGHAN L.C. (1972) The use of bone autografts in canine orthopaedic surgery. *J. small Anim. Pract.* **13,** 455.

VAUGHAN L.C. (1975) Complications associated with the internal fixation of fractures in dogs. *J. small Anim. Pract.* **16,** 415.

VAUGHAN L.C. & Robins G.M. (1975) Surgical remodelling of the femoral trochlea: an experimental study. *Vet. Rec.* **96,** 447.

WALTER J.B. & ISRAEL M.S. (1967) *General Pathology.* J. & A. Churchill Ltd, London, Toronto.

WEBER H. & CECH O. (1976) *Pseudoarthrosis.* Bern, H. Huber, Verlag.

WOLFF J. (1892) *Das Gesetz der Transformation der Knochen.* A. Hirschwald, Berlin.

Chapter 2
The Treatment of Fractures

Once a fracture has been reduced, and provided the blood supply to the fragments is intact, the main requirement for successful healing is the provision of adequate immobilization (see page 7).

Each fracture should be considered in terms of its inherent stability or resistance to shortening, angulation and rotation when choosing the appropriate fixation technique. On this basis, fractures can be divided into:

Stable fractures (Fig. 32a)
Transverse or greenstick fractures, where the fragments interlock and resist shortening. Here fixation is needed to prevent angular deformity only. A cast can be used when this type of fracture occurs below the elbow or stifle while an intramedullary pin is often effective when the fracture involves the humerus or the femur.

Unstable fractures (Fig. 32b)
Oblique, spiral or comminuted fractures. Here the fragments do not interlock, fixation is needed to maintain

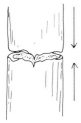

Fragments interlock
and resist shortening
Fixation needed to prevent angular
deformity

Fig. 32a. Stable fractures—transverse or greenstick.

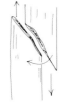

Fragments do not interlock
Fixation needed to maintain length,
alignment and prevent rotation...

Fig. 32b. Unstable fractures—oblique, spiral or comminuted.

35

length, alignment and prevent rotation. Intramedullary pinning provides poor resistance against these forces unless used in combination with cerclage wire in oblique or spiral fractures. The ideal method for this group of unstable fractures is to use lag screws in combination with a plate. The main methods of fracture fixation commonly in use are briefly described below.

Closed reduction and external fixation of fractures using splints or casts

1   The joint above and below the fracture must be immobilized, therefore the method is usually limited to fractures *below* the elbow and the stifle. However, it is possible to immobilize the humerus or femur with a Thomas extension splint (Fig. 33d). Alternatively, a body cast may be used for

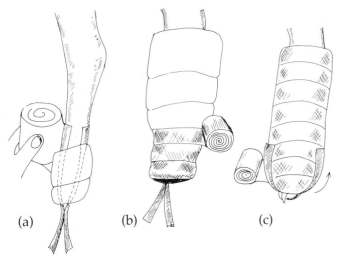

(a) (b) (c)

Fig. 33a. Elastoplast strips are placed down the anterior and posterior aspect of the foot (these will prevent the bandage slipping off the leg) and can be used for traction during application of the cotton wool layers.

Fig. 33b. A 1 pound roll of cotton wool is split into 2 narrower ½ pound rolls and these are used to pad the leg. The total amount of cotton wool required ranges from ½ to 2 lb depending on the size of the dog.

Fig. 33c
The ends of the elastoplast tape are flapped back to reveal the pads of the foot and then attached to the end of the bandage using elastoplast.
The cotton wool is tightly compressed with a Vetwrap elasticated bandage.

36

the humerus (Fig. 34a).

2   External fixation is most effective for fractures with inherent stability—i.e. transverse or oblique fractures of less than 45°.

3   After closed reduction, radiographs should be taken to ensure that at least 50% of the fracture surfaces are in contact.

First aid procedures for temporary immobilization of fractures or injured joints

ROBERT JONES BANDAGE

The Robert Jones bandage is a thick cotton wool bandage which provides immobilization and controls oedema. For these reasons it is useful not only as a first aid measure for the temporary immobilization of fractures but also as a post–operative bandage for fractures which have been treated surgically. The bandage is comfortable to wear and is generally well tolerated despite its bulk.

Application (Figs. 33a,b,c)

THE THOMAS EXTENSION SPLIT

Although this splint can be used as the sole method of fixation for stable fractures below the elbow or stifle, it is generally only used as a temporary splint for limb bone fractures. The splint is usually constructed from aluminium rod, however coat hanger wire can be used in small dogs.

A ring is made in the rod to fit round the base of the leg (Fig. 33d (i), (ii)).

The base of the ring is bent in at an angle to avoid pressure on the femoral blood vessels and the ring is padded with cotton wool (Fig. 33d (iii)). The splint is pushed firmly into the inguinal region and the cranial bar of the splint is bent to conform to the leg's normal angulation in the standing position (Fig. 33d (iv)). Elastoplast strips are used to fix the foot to the end of the bar. The upper part of the leg is also attached to the cranial bar with elastoplast, while a thick band of elastoplast is placed round both bars and the hock (Fig. 33d (v)).

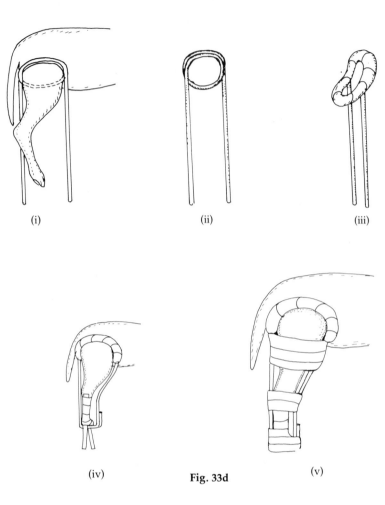

(i)
(ii)
(iii)

(iv)
Fig. 33d
(v)

VELPEAU SLING BANDAGE (Figs 33e (i), (ii), (iii))
This bandage is used to immobilize shoulder and scapular injuries and to prevent weight bearing. A conforming gauze bandage is wrapped around the paw, the leg is flexed and the bandage is brought up over the lateral aspect of the shoulder and around the chest. Several layers are applied and then covered with elastoplast.

EHMER SLING (Fig. 33f)
The Ehmer sling prevents weight bearing on the hind leg and its main use is to provide partial immobilization of the

38

hip following reduction of a dislocation.

The casting materials used today include:
1   Plaster of Paris.
2   Vetcast (Scotchcast from 3M)—fibreglass.
3   Baycast (Bayer UK Ltd).
4   Hexcelite (HEXCEL medical products).
Plaster of Paris remains one of the most popular casting materials because it is easy to apply and readily conforms to the shape of the limb. However, plaster is heavy and lacks strength compared with the newer casting materials such as Vetcast or Baycast.

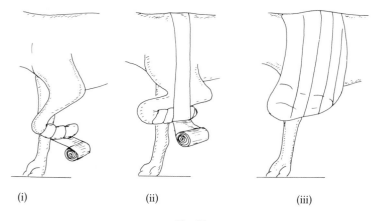

(i)   (ii)   (iii)

Fig. 33e

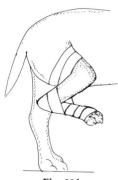

Fig. 33f

39

Application of a plaster of Paris cast to immobilize an undisplaced transverse fracture of the radius and ulna

1   The dog should be anaesthetized for application of the cast.

2   Strips of elastoplast are applied down the anterior and posterior aspects of the leg and these can be used to exert traction on the limb during application of the cast (Fig. 33g (i)).

3   A stockinet is applied to the limb, this should extend from below the toes to well above the elbow (Fig. 33g (ii)).

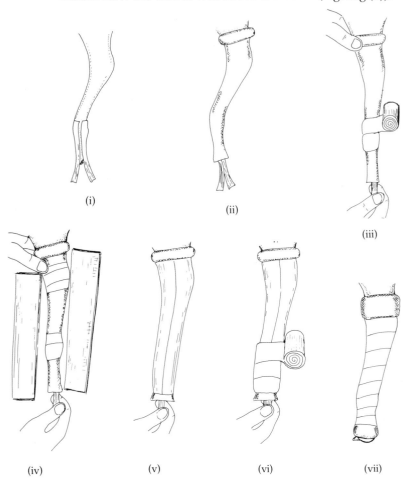

(i)

(ii)

(iii)

(iv)

(v)

(vi)

(vii)

Fig. 33g (i–vii). Application of a Plaster of Paris cast to immobilize the forearm.

40

4   Two or three layers of cast padding (Soffban [Smith & Nephew]) are applied next starting from the toes and working up to the elbow (Fig. 33g (iii)).

5   An assistant holds the leg in extension, one hand is used to steady the leg above the elbow while the other exerts traction on the elastoplast foot tapes (Fig. 33g (iv)). Two slabs of plaster of Paris are prepared, they should be 4 layers thick and of sufficient length to extend from above the elbow to the foot (Fig. 33g (iv)). The slabs are soaked in lukewarm water and then applied to the anterior and posterior aspect of the leg. Next, run your hands up and down the cast to ensure the slabs are evenly applied and conform to the shape of the leg (Fig. 33g (v)). Take a roll of plaster of Paris, hold on to the free end and dunk the roll into water till it is thoroughly saturated, i.e. till all the air bubbles have stopped coming out of it. Squeeze excess water from the plaster and apply it over the slabs in a wrapround fashion starting from the foot and working up the leg (Fig. 33g (vi)). Finally, fold back the stockinet at the top and bottom of the cast together with the foot tags and stick these down with a little more plaster of Paris (Fig. 33g (vii)). It is important that the stockinet at the distal end of the cast is folded back sufficiently for the pads to be exposed so that they can be checked regularly to ensure that the circulation to the foot has not been compromised. Although plaster of Paris sets rapidly the cast will take at least 8 hours to dry out. Once it has dried out several layers of elastoplast are used to protect it. The cast is changed at 2 weeks when soft tissue swelling will have subsided. The second cast is left on for 4 weeks or longer till sufficient callus has developed to immobilize the fracture.

The cast should be inspected by a veterinary surgeon at least once a week. The owner should feel the cast each day to check that it feels warm and is not rubbing. The pads should also be checked daily to ensure the circulation to the foot is not being compromised. Warn the owner that if the cast begins to smell or the dog starts to chew frantically at the cast, stops putting weight on the leg or goes off his food, veterinary attention must be sought immediately and the cast changed.

External skeletal fixation using the Kirshner splint (AO/ASIF External skeletal fixator)—Straumann, Great Britain Ltd).

The method involves the transcutaneous insertion of 2 half pins each in the proximal and distal bone segments, which are then connected by an external bar. Generally, the splint is placed on the craniolateral surface of the humerus, the craniomedial surface of the radius, the lateral surface of the femur and the medial surface of the tibia.

The Kirshner splint is ideal for the treatment of compound or infected fractures because the half pins can be inserted into healthy bone at some distance from the fracture site. The method is also useful for stabilizing corrective osteotomies. The treatment of a tibial shaft fracture using the AO/ASIF External skeletal fixator is shown in Fig. 34b. The device is well tolerated provided it is properly applied.

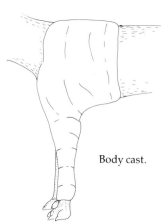

Body cast.

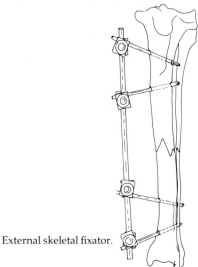

Fig. 34.

External skeletal fixator.

Open reduction and internal fixation of fractures

The indications for open reduction and internal fixation are:
1 Fractures that cannot be treated by closed methods.
2 Unstable fractures—comminuted or oblique.
3 Fractures involving articular surfaces where accurate anatomical reduction is essential.
4 Avulsion fractures.

42

1   Intramedullary pins.
2   Wire–sutures
        –cerclage
        –tension band.
3   Lag screws
4   Plates and screws.

Intramedullary pins

An intramedullary pin is a metal rod which is inserted into the medullary cavity of a bone to maintain reduction of a fracture. Although the pin disturbs endosteal callus formation it causes little interference with the healing of the cortex and periosteum of the bone. Primary bone union should occur when the pin tightly impacts the medullary cavity and completely immobilizes the fracture, whereas marked periosteal callus formation occurs when a loose fitting pin is used for fixation. Biomechanical studies have shown that bone is stronger after fracture healing when an intramedullary pin has been used for fixation as opposed to a plate (Braden *et al* 1973). This is related to a phenomenon called 'stress protection' and is discussed further on page 65.

THE CRITERIA FOR INTRAMEDULLARY FIXATION ARE:
1   Shaft fractures of long bones such as the femur which are relatively straight and have a medullary cavity of uniform diameter.
2   Relatively transverse fractures which will impact under weight bearing.
    The main disadvantage of the intramedullary pin is that rotational stability is poor. However this is outweighed by advantages such as:
1   Ease and speed of insertion and removal of the pin.
2   Low cost.
3   The intramedullary pin is a stronger method of fixation than the plate, and bone is also stronger following fracture healing when this method is used.
4   A pin which crosses an epiphyseal plate causes minimal

disturbance in bone growth when compared with other methods of internal fixation.

There are three types of intramedullary pin:
1   The Steinman pin.
2   The Kuntscher nail.
3   The Rush pin.

STEINMAN PIN

The Steinman pin is the pin most frequently used in veterinary orthopaedics and little specialist equipment is needed for its insertion (Figs. 35–38).

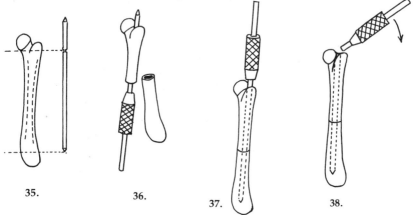

35.

36.

37.

38.

Fig. 35. Pin measured against a radiograph of the normal femur and pre-cut.
Fig. 36. Pin introduced into proximal shaft of femur in a retrograde manner using a chuck, pin emerges in trochanteric fossa.
Fig. 37. Position of chuck reversed, fracture reduced, pin driven down into distal shaft of femur.
Fig. 38. Pin broken off flush in trochanteric fossa.

Equipment (Arnolds Ltd)
1   Intramedullary pin insertor with Jacobs chuck.
2   Selection of Steinman pins (1/16 in to 1/4 in diameter, 7 in–12 in in length).
3   Stainless steel wire (18, 20 and 24 gauge).
4   Hacksaw, wire cutters, wire twisters, pin cutters.
5   Two pairs of bone holding forceps.
    The use of a Steinman pin for fixation of a fractured femur is illustrated in Figs 35–38.

44

In large dogs it may be necessary to insert two or three Steinman pins to fill the medullary cavity. Provided the pin has been broken off below the tip of the greater trochanter and remains in this position it can be left *in situ* after healing is complete. In immature dogs rapid longitudinal growth of the bone often seals the pin within the diaphysis. However in mature dogs there is a tendency for the pin to migrate dorsally ('ride up') and cause soft tissue damage. In this event the pin is removed provided that fracture healing is complete. Some surgeons prefer to remove all intramedullary pins and use a longer pin which is cut off just below the skin surface to allow for easy removal.

THE KUNTSCHER NAIL

The Kuntscher nail (Kuntscher 1965) is a clover leaf or V-shaped hollow nail (Fig. 39). It is available in diameters ranging from 2 mm–20 mm and in any length required. One end of the nail is sharpened for impaction and at the other end there is a hole to engage an extractor hook.

Equipment for insertion of the nail is relatively expensive when compared with that for Steinman pins. The use of nails has been limited in canine orthopaedics to transverse shaft fractures of the femur and to a lesser extent humeral

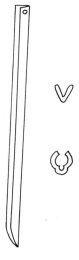

Fig. 39. Kuntscher nail.

45

fractures. The nail is inserted at the extremity of the bone and then driven down the medullary cavity. The shape of the Kuntscher nail ensures a good grip in cancellous bone and provided a nail is selected which tightly impacts the medullary cavity, rotation at the fracture site is kept to a minimum.

THE RUSH PIN

The design of the Rush pin is illustrated in Fig. 41. The pin has a pointed 'sledge runner' tip for ease of insertion while the other end is hooked to ensure good fixation and simplify removal. The pins are available in various sizes with diameters ranging from 5/32–1/4 in and lengths from 1 in–17 in.

The Rush pin immobilizes the fracture by its spring-like action which results in three-point pressure within the medullary cavity (Fig. 43). This method of fixation is most commonly used for supracondylar fractures of the femur and humerus. Two pins are used and the mode of insertion is illustrated in Figs 40–43.

The use of two Rush pins for fixation of a supracondylar fracture of the femur

The fracture is reduced and an awl-reamer or Steinman pin is used to penetrate the cortex of the distal fragment to allow insertion of the Rush pin. The angle of insertion should be 30–40° to the long axis of the bone (Fig. 40). The first Rush pin is introduced and used to maintain reduction of the fracture (Fig. 41); the second Rush pin is introduced (Fig. 42).

Once the fracture is correctly held in alignment the pins are hammered alternatively until each is seated and the hook head grips the cortex.

Orthopaedic wire

Orthopaedic wire is made of monofilament stainless steel and is available in sizes ranging from 18–28 gauge. 18 gauge wire is the thickest and has a diameter of 1.2 mm.

Wire sutures may be used as the sole method of fixation

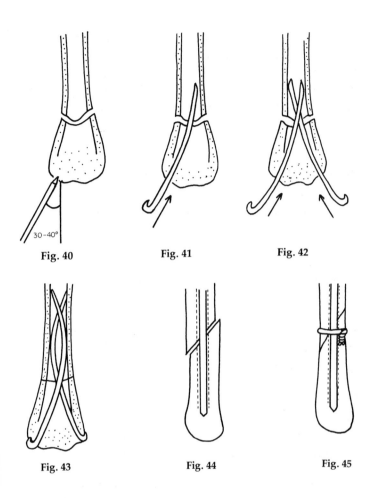

Fig. 40

Fig. 41

Fig. 42

Fig. 43

Fig. 44

Fig. 45

particularly in fractures of the mandible and skull. Simple interrupted sutures are used to retain the fragments in place. A straight traumatic needle serves as a cheap substitute for a small diameter drill bit to drill holes through the fragments through which the wire is threaded.

Wire is frequently used in combination with intramedullary pins for fracture fixation, either to retain fragments in alignment or to provide rotational stability. If an intramedullary pin is used as the sole method of fixation for an oblique midshaft fracture of the femur, the fragments tend to override and there may be rotation at the fracture site.

A simple way to overcome this problem is to supplement the pin with a 360° cerclage wire (Fig. 45).

The 360° cerclage wire however is a controversial method of fixation. It has been condemned by some (Newton & Hohn 1974; Vaughan 1975) as it is said to cause non–union by interference with the periosteal blood supply. Others (Withrow & Holmberg 1977) favour cerclage and attribute failures of the method to poor case selection and poor technical application rather than interference with blood supply. Normal bone receives blood from a variety of sources, these include: the nutrient artery, the metaphyseal vessels and fascial attachments to the periosteum. If the blood supply in cortical bone was longitudinal to the long axis, then this could be 'strangled' by a cerclage wire, however, this is not the case. Vascular supply within the cortical bone is perpendicular rather than longitudinal to the long axis and it has been shown (Cohen & Harris 1958) that the longitudinal vascular supply is limited to one or two millimetres. Consequently when 2 cerclage wires are used to stabilize an oblique fracture (Fig. 46) the segment of bone between them does not become necrotic. It is vascularized initially and in a centripedal fashion by vessels arising from the surrounding soft tissues and the periosteum. As healing progresses the normal centrifugal blood flow within the haversion systems will be restored.

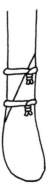

Fig. 46

The proper application of cerclage wires should result in compression of the fracture and primary bone union will often occur. Conversely, a loose cerclage wire results in resorption of bone or lysis under the wire and leads to non–union of the fracture. The potential for bone necrosis may be exacerbated by excessive periosteal stripping and poor standards of asepsis.

360° cerclage wire should be reserved for oblique or spiral shaft fractures. 18 gauge (1.2 mm diameter) wire is used for animals over 20 kg while at least 20 gauge (1 mm diameter) wire is used for animals under 20 kg. The wire should be applied tightly and specific wire tighteners are available for this purpose (Fig. 47). The wire is tied either by twisting (Fig. 48) or by use of an ASIF loop (Fig. 49).

If a twist knot is used, it is important to ensure that the first few twists are equally distributed on each wire (Fig. 48). Uneven twisting may cause the wire to break before it is fully tightened or the formation of a slip knot (Fig. 50) which may loosen.

Movement of a cerclage wire can cause lysis of the under-lying bone. This complication can be minimized by ensuring that the wire is applied tightly and if necessary the

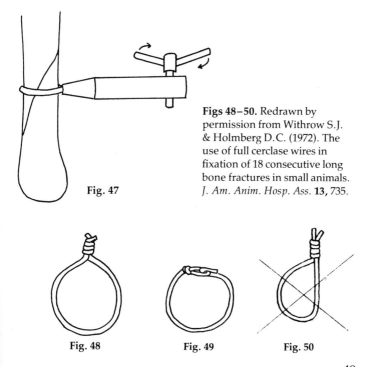

Figs 48–50. Redrawn by permission from Withrow S.J. & Holmberg D.C. (1972). The use of full cerclase wires in fixation of 18 consecutive long bone fractures in small animals. *J. Am. Anim. Hosp. Ass.* **13,** 735.

Fig. 47

Fig. 48   Fig. 49   Fig. 50

cortex of the bone is notched to prevent the wire slipping. However, if absolute stability is to be ensured, the wire should penetrate the cortex of the bone (Fig. 51a and b) before it is passed round the fragments.

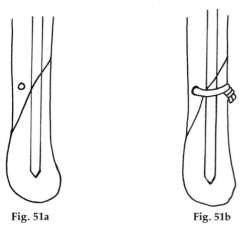

Fig. 51a   Fig. 51b

Wire may also be used in combination with pins or alone as a wire tension band to compress a fracture site. The application of this method of fixation is described on page 58.

Bone plates

The correct application of a bone plate and screws should result in optimal stability at the fracture site and allow early painfree limb function.

There has been considerable interest in the use of compression plates during the past 15 years. Although there is a definite role for this type of plate in veterinary orthopaedics, especially large animal work, the equipment is very expensive. In the dog good results can be obtained using the cheaper traditional plates and self-tapping screws for fracture fixation. These plates are applied without compression and include:

1   *The Sherman plate* (Fig. 52). This is a weak plate and its use is mainly limited to small dogs.

2   *The Lane bone plate* (Fig. 53). This is similar to the Sherman plate but far weaker.

50

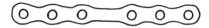

Fig. 52. Sherman plate.

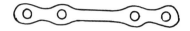

Fig. 53. Lane plate.

3   *The Venables bone plate* (Fig. 54). There are no con-
strictions between the screw holes and consequently the
plate is strong and ideal for general veterinary orthopaedics. A heavy duty Venables plate is also available, and
can be used in very large dogs.

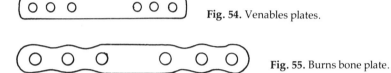

Fig. 54. Venables plates.

Fig. 55. Burns bone plate.

4   *The Burns bone plate* (Fig. 55). This is a modification of
both the Sherman and Venables type plates. It combines the
attributes of both—i.e. strength and reduction in the size of
the implant.
5   *Finger plates* are also available for fracture fixation in
miniature dogs.
   The Sherman screw is the standard orthopaedic screw
and is self-tapping a 9/64ths in diameter screw is suitable for
most dogs.

APPLICATIONS OF A BONE PLATE
Insertion of a bone plate using 9/64 in diameter Sherman
screws is illustrated in Figs 56–59.
   The fracture is reduced and the longest plate that can be
easily inserted is chosen. This should allow at least 2 screws

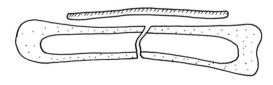

Fig. 56

to be placed on either side of the fracture to provide satisfactory immobilization. The plate is accurately contoured to the shape of the bone using plate benders.

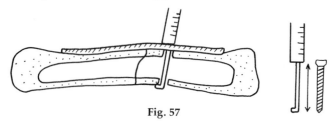

Fig. 57

A 7/64 in bit is used to drill the first screw hole about 1 cm from the fracture site. The hole should penetrate both cortices. A depth gauge is used to measure the length of the hole and a screw chosen of that length. The screw thread should grip in both cortices.

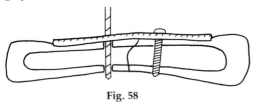

Fig. 58

After insertion of the first screw, the next screw hole is drilled on the other side of the fracture site. The appropriate screw is inserted.

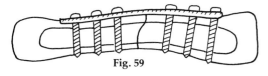

Fig. 59

The rest of the screws are inserted working away from the fracture site.

The weakest point on any plate is the screw hole and care should be taken in the application of a plate to avoid leaving an empty screw hole directly over the fracture site, otherwise the plate may break at this point before healing is complete. If it is only possible to insert one screw in the distal fragment then external support must be provided. Occasionally the screw thread that has been cut in the bone

52

is stripped and under these circumstances the screw cannot be tightened. The screw should be removed and replaced by one of a larger diameter (5/32ths). The indications for plate removal are given on page 65.

EQUIPMENT FOR PLATING
(Arnolds or Zimmer G. Britain Ltd)
Hand drill—drill bits 7/64 in and 9/64 in.
Depth gauge.
Ruler.
Zimmer screwdriver.
Burns bone holding forceps ×2.
Bone clamp for small bones ×2.
Plate benders.
Burns plates.
Venables plates.
Selection of screws 1/2 in to 2 in (9/64 in diameter).
Bone cutters.
Chisel.
Gouge.

The use of compression in the treatment of fractures— ASIF methods (Muller *et al* 1970)

In 1958 a group of Swiss surgeons, engineers and metal-lurgists formed an association to study internal fixation for fresh fractures and for non–union fractures of long bones. They called themselves the AO group (Arbeitsgemeinschaft fuer Osteosynthesefragan). More recently they have be-come known as the Association for the Study of Internal Fixation (ASIF). The chief aim of the ASIF method is to restore full function to the injured limb as quickly as pos-sible (Muller *et al* 1969).
   This is achieved by:
1   Atraumatic surgical technique.
2   Accurate anatomical reduction especially in intra-articular fractures.
3   Rigid internal fixation.
4   The avoidance of soft tissue damage and fracture disease, i.e. joint stiffness, muscle wasting and osteo-porosis by early mobilization.

Rigid internal fixation of a fracture can be achieved by compression or intramedullary nailing (page 45) and should result in primary bone union (page 7).

Compression may be:
1 Interfragmental.
2 Axial.
3 A combination of 1 and 2.

(page 45)

INTERFRAGMENTAL COMPRESSION

Interfragmental compression is a method of compressing two fragments of bone together and is achieved by the lag screw principle. This is illustrated in Figs 60, 61 and 62. The

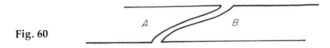

Fig. 60

method of drilling holes depends on the type of screw used but basically if fragment A is to be lagged to fragment B using a screw (Fig. 60), then the hole in fragment A must be

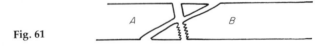

Fig. 61

large enough for the screw to pass through it without the thread getting a grip (gliding hole). The screw thread must only grip in the far cortex of fragment B (Fig. 61).

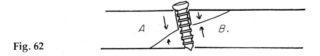

Fig. 62

As the screw is tightened interfragmentary compression results (Fig. 62). If the screw thread gripped in both cortices it would be impossible to compress the fracture.

ASIF bone screws are made with a much larger area of thread contact surface at more nearly rightangles to the long axis of the screw than is present in most conventional bone screws, and this ensures a full grip in the bone. In addition a tap is used to cut a thread in the bone. This ensures a good

54

fit for the screw thread without damage to the bone. If an ASIF bone screw of incorrect length is inserted it can be removed and replaced with another without risk of damage to the thread in the bone. Self-tapping screws on the other hand give rise to multiple microfractures as they are inserted. The result is fibrous tissue formation around the thread which offers the screw a poor hold in the bone.

Two types of ASIF bone screws have been developed, the cortex screw (Fig. 63) for use in the hard cortical bone of the

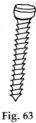

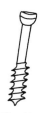

Fig. 63

Fig. 64

Cortex screws are available in the following diameters:*
1.5 mm (drill bit 1.1 mm)
2.0 mm (,, ,, 1.5 mm)
2.7 mm (,, ,, 2.0 mm)
3.5 mm (,, ,, 2.5 mm)
4.5 mm (,, ,, 3.2 mm)
    *Synthes, Straumann (Great Britain) Ltd.

Cancellous screws are available in the following diameters:*
4.0 mm (drill bit 2.0 mm)
6.5 mm (,, ,, 3.2 mm)

diaphysis, and the cancellous screw (Fig. 64) for use in the soft cancellous bone of the metaphysis and epiphysis, this screw has a coarser thread for this purpose.

When cancellous screws are used for the fixation of condylar fractures it is not necessary to enlarge the hole in the proximal fragment provided the thread grips in the far fragment only (Figs 65 and 66).

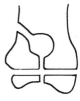

Fig. 65

Fig. 66

Interfragmental compression using screws alone can be employed for oblique or spiral fractures of the diaphysis when the length of the fracture is four times the diameter of the shaft (Fig. 67). The angle of insertion of lag screws is of some importance.

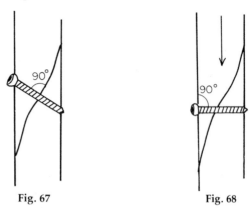

Fig. 67   Fig. 68

In an oblique fracture a screw at right angles to the fracture line will give maximum interfragmental compression (Fig. 67); while a screw placed at right angles to the shaft would offer maximum resistance to shortening but not complete interfragmental compression (Fig. 68). Maximum use of the good qualities shown in Figs 67 and 68 can be made by insertion of the screw along an imaginary line that bisects the angle between a perpendicular to the long axis of the shaft and a perpendicular to the fracture plane (Fig. 69). In practice several screws are inserted at different angles to each other to counteract shearing and torsional forces and at

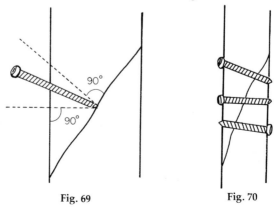

Fig. 69   Fig. 70

least one of the screws is placed at right angles to the long axis of the bone (Fig. 70).

When screws are used as the sole method of internal fixation for a shaft fracture then external support with a plaster cast should also be provided.

AXIAL COMPRESSION

Whenever possible axial compression is achieved by employing the tension band principle (Pauwels 1965) and this is illustrated in Figs 71–74.

If a bone is thought of as a column, and a load is placed over its centre (Fig. 71) then within the column there are only compressive forces. However, if the load is placed on one side of the column (Fig. 72) then there are extra bending or compressive forces exerted on this side of the column with equal and opposite tensile forces on the other side of the column. These tensile forces can be neutralized with a tension band which is shown as a chain in Fig. 73. It acts as if a load had been placed on this side of the column giving compression as in Fig. 74.

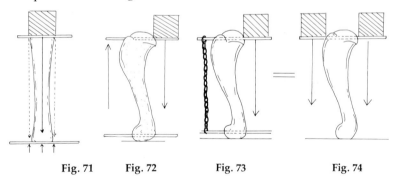

Fig. 71   Fig. 72   Fig. 73   Fig. 74

Normally bones are unevenly loaded so that one side of the bone is under compression and another side under tension. Implants should be placed on the tension side of the bone otherwise they will be subjected to repeated bending and compressive forces and may break before fracture healing is complete (Figs 74a and b). Unfortunately the loading of bone is not as simple as shown in Figs. 71–74b. The stresses in bone are continually changing depending on:

(a) weight bearing.
(b) locomotion.
(c) muscle pull.

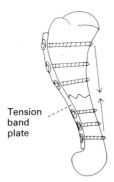

Fig. 74a. Apply implant on the tension side.

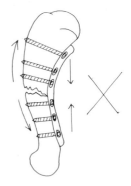

Fig. 74b. If applied to compression side, excessive bending results in plate fracture.

A fracture causes a total disruption in the normal stresses. Nevertheless the tension side of certain long bones has been established, i.e.

The proximal anterior humerus.

The caudal aspect of the olecranon.

The proximal lateral femur.

The antero-medial aspect of the distal tibia.

Although a plate should be placed on the tensile side of a bone whenever possible, this consideration takes third priority in the list shown below:

Plate position:

1   On aspect of bone which is easiest to expose.

2   Consider position of lag screws in relation to the plate and choice of exposure.

3   Place on tensile side of bone if possible.

AXIAL COMPRESSION USING A WIRE TENSION BAND

This method is used for treatment of avulsion fractures of the olecranon, greater trochanter, patella, tibial crest, and and os calcis. In all these fractures the fragment is distracted by the muscle, tendon or ligament which inserts on it. The tension band is placed so that it counteracts the tensile force

58

acting on the fragment and redirects it to compress the fragment against the adjacent bone (Pauwels 1965).

Avulsion of the tibial crest is used as an example. This is a fairly common injury in the immature Greyhound and the fracture occurs through the growth plate. The tibial crest is distracted by the tensile force of the quadriceps muscle exerted through the straight patellar ligament (Fig. 75). The fracture is reduced and initial fixation is achieved with 2 Kirschner wires driven through the crest into the metaphysis (Fig. 76). A hole is drilled transversely through the

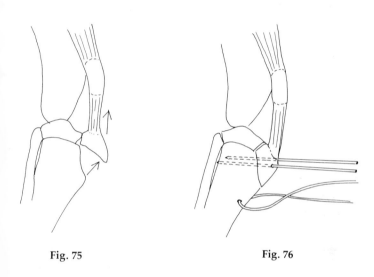

Fig. 75   Fig. 76

tibia distal to the fracture site (Fig. 76). A length of stainless steel wire (20 gauge) is passed through the hole, the ends of the wire are brought across the anterior aspect of the tibia in a figure of 8 pattern and then passed through the straight patellar ligament before being twisted tight (Fig. 77a,b,c). As the wire is tightened (Fig. 77a) its proximal loop engages on the protruding ends of the Kirschner wires (Fig. 77a). Each Kirschner wire is then bent (Fig. 77a) and cut leaving a hook about 1/2 cm long which is rotated up to fit snugly with the tibial crest and insertion of the straight patellar ligament (Fig. 77b). The implants can be left in situ once fracture healing is complete unless the ends of the wires cause soft tissue damage which necessitates their removal.

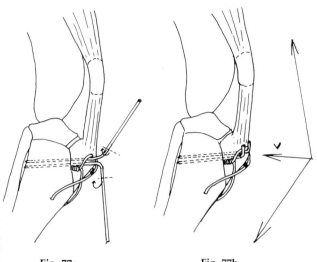

Fig. 77a   Fig. 77b

The wire tension band counteracts the pull of the straight patellar ligament and the resultant vector (v) compresses the fracture site (Fig. 77b). The tension band is acting in exactly the same way as a guy rope holding up a tent pole (Fig. 78). Imagine the tent pole is the tibial crest, the straight patellar ligament is one guy rope and the tension

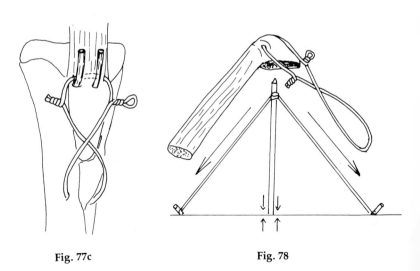

Fig. 77c   Fig. 78

band wire is the other. The opposing pull of the two guy ropes will cause compression between the tent pole and the ground or, in this example, between the tibial crest and the metaphysis.

Whenever a plate is used to compress a fracture it is in fact acting as a tension band because the plate must be placed under tension to give compression. Tension in the plate is achieved either with a tension device (see Figs. 79–81) or by displacement of the plate through eccentrically placed screws (see Figs 85–9).

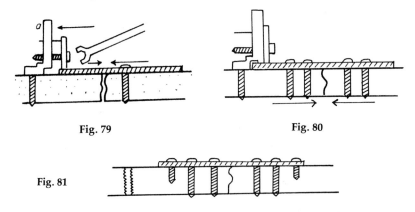

Fig. 79   Fig. 80

Fig. 81

AXIAL COMPRESSION USING PLATES

Axial compression using a plate and a tension device
This method is illustrated in Figs 79–81. It requires large exposure and its use is basically confined to fractures of the proximal or distal third of long bones.

The fracture is reduced (Fig. 79), a plate is applied and a

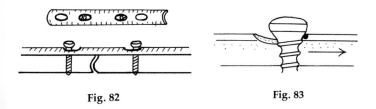

Fig. 82   Fig. 83

Figs 82–84 Redrawn by permission of Muller M.E., Allgower M. & Willneger H. (1970). *Manual of Internal Fixation.* Springer Verlag, Berlin, Heidelberg, New York.

screw inserted approximately 1 cm from the fracture site. The tension device *a* is then attached to the plate and screwed to the bone.

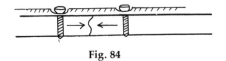

Fig. 84

The tension device is tightened to compress the fracture (Fig. 80), the remaining screws are inserted and the device is removed. When possible to ensure that there is a gradual gradient between rigid bone under the plate and normal elastic bone the end screw is placed through one cortex only; this helps avoid the risk of re-fracture at the end of the plate.

Figs 85–89. Redrawn by permission of Allgower M., Matter P., Perren S.M. & Ruedi T. (1973). The dynamic compression plate (DCP). Springer Verlag, Berlin, Heidelberg, New York.

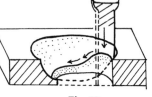

Fig. 85

Axial compression using a semi-tubular plate
In many circumstances it is not possible to use a tension device to compress fractures and this led to the development of plates with screw holes that permitted a self-compressing action. The two types of plate with this feature are the semi-tubular plate and the dynamic compression plate (DCP).

The screw is placed eccentrically (i.e. at one end of the oval screw hole, Figs 82 and 83). The conical geometry of the screw shoulder against the oval screw hole of the plate, Fig. 83, ensures that as the screw is tightened the plate is placed under tension and the fracture is compressed.

The semi-tubular plate is light and its shape ensures a good fit on the underlying bone. It should only be used on the tension side of a bone as it has poor resistance to bending.

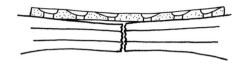

Fig. 86

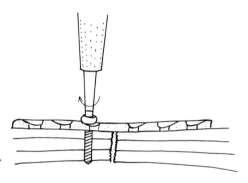

Fig. 87

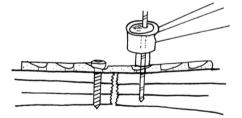

Fig. 88

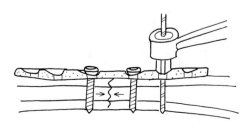

Fig. 89

The dynamic compression plate (Allgower *et al* 1973).

The main feature of the ᴅᴄᴘ is the design of the screw hole which is based on the spherical gliding principle. This enables the ᴅᴄᴘ to be used as a self-compressing plate. Insertion of the screw will displace the plate resulting in compression of the fracture as the screw head is tightened against the hemicylindrical slope of the screw hole (Fig. 85).

The spherical geometry of the screw hole also ensures that there is a congruent fit between the screw and the plate in any position along the screw hole, while permitting a certain degree of tilt between the screw and the plate.

The ᴅᴄᴘ is ideal for treating multiple fractures of a long bone in that individual fragments can be compressed together by the introduction of successive screws in the plate.

The application of the ᴅᴄᴘ as a self-compressing plate is illustrated in Figs 86 to 89. The fracture is reduced and the plate carefully contoured to fit the bone (Fig. 86). The plate is then secured to one of the main fragments by means of a screw inserted about 1 cm from the fracture site. A neutral guide is used for positioning the screw (Fig. 87). The second screw is placed in the opposite fragment but with the aid of the loaded drill guide, as this screw is tightened the fracture is compressed (Fig. 88). The remaining screws are inserted with the aid of the neutral drill guide (Fig. 89).

The neutralization plate

This means the use of any plate without compression (especially for comminuted fractures) to transmit all

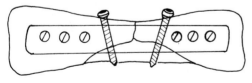

Fig. 90i. Neutralization plate.

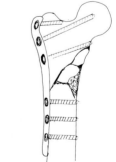

Fig. 90ii. Buttress plate.

torsional and bending forces from the proximal to the distal fragment of a bone and thus prevent these forces acting on fracture surfaces which have been stabilized by inter-fragmental compression using lag screws (Fig. 90i).

Buttress plate

If a plate is used to shore up a fragment of bone or to span an area of comminution where fragments are too small for lag screw fixation then the plate is said to function as a buttress plate (Fig. 90ii).

The indications for plate removal

Normally there is no need to remove plates which have been used to stabilize fractures in middle-aged dogs. Plates that have been used for fixation of the jaw and pelvis in dogs of any age are also left *in situ* after healing is complete.

When plates are used in the treatment of long bone frac-tures in dogs under three years of age, particularly working dogs, it is usual to remove the plate after three to four months to avoid the phenomenon of 'stress protection'. Normal bone is constantly subjected to mechanical stresses that result in some bone deformation or strain every time weight is put on it or when isotonic contraction of muscle occurs. These constantly changing stresses seem to be essential for the maintenance of the functional architecture of bone. When a rigid plate is used for fracture fixation the underlying bone is protected from stress (Allgower *et al* 1969). According to Wolff's law of adaption to functional demand this stress protection will cause bone destruction to prevail over osteogenesis in the course of remodelling lead-ing to osteoporosis and a risk of refracture at one or other end of the plate. Stress protection depends on the rigidity of the plate inserted and fortunately this phenomenon is rare in dogs provided implants of the correct size are used (Brinker *et al* 1977).

Although it is desirable to remove the plates after healing of long bone fractures in young dogs, in the case of the humerus it is often safer to leave the plate *in situ* to avoid iatrogenic damage to the radial nerve. (It is often difficult to identify the nerve during exposure of the plate through the development of scar tissue from the initial open reduction).

Other indications for plate removal are when fracture healing is complicated by infection and osteomyelitis or when a plate crosses a growth plate in an immature animal. Rejection of plates and screws due to corrosion or foreign body reaction has now become a rare occurrence as materials used in the manufacture of these implants are of high quality.

When a plate is used for fixation of fractures of the radius or tibia there is little soft tissue cover. This sometimes leads to skin reactions over the plate or lameness due to temperature changes between the plate and bone and under these circumstances the implant should be removed.

Growth plate injuries

Local disorders of bone growth form an important group of orthopaedic problems that occur in dogs. A typical long bone is developed from three primary centres of ossification, one for the diaphysis and one for each epiphysis. In many bones secondary centres are also present and it is from these that various processes such as the tuberosities develop. Longitudinal growth of bone occurs from the growth plate, a zone of cartilage interposed between the diaphysis and epiphysis. The cells of the growth plate are shown in diagrammatic form in Fig. 90a. Closest to the epiphysis are the germinal or resting cartilage cells; these give rise to a zone of proliferating young cartilage cells. Then there is a zone of hypertrophic cartilage cells, the matrix between the cells is scanty. This zone is the weak link in the growth plate. In a traumatic epiphyseal separation (epiphysiolysis) cleavage occurs through the zone of hypertrophic cartilage cells. This is of clinical importance because the germinal cells remain with the epiphysis so there is still potential for longitudinal growth of bone after reduction of the separation. Proceeding into the metaphysis from the growth plate the cartilage calcifies and undergoes enchondral ossification.

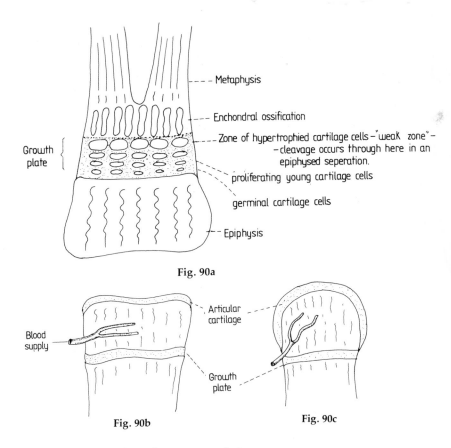

Fig. 90a

Fig. 90b

Fig. 90c

Growth plate disorders can result from:

1 Trauma—a fracture or crush injury or a disruption of blood supply to the germinal cells.

2 Bridging of the growth plate with a metal implant will eventually cause premature closure of the growth plate. Implants should be removed within 4 weeks if growth is to continue.

The blood supply to the epiphysis influences the prognosis following epiphyseal separation. Fortunately most epiphyses have the type of blood shown in Fig. 90b and this remains intact despite displacement. However, if the epiphysis is covered by articular cartilage (Fig. 90c) as for example the capital femoral epiphysis, then blood vessels can only enter at the perichondrium and these will be disrupted when separation occurs, leading to avascular necrosis of the epiphysis.

Salter and Harris (1963), have classified growth plate injuries into 6 types:

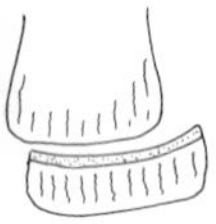

Type 1. Separation without fracture. After realignment healing is rapid and the prognosis is good. The exception is separation of the capital femoral epiphysis. (See above).

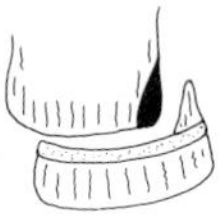

Type 2. This is the most common. Separation of the epiphysis occurs associated with fracture of a triangular piece of the metaphysis. Provided accurate reduction is carried out the prognosis is good.

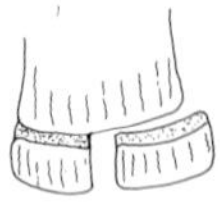

Type 3. This type is uncommon. It is seen near the end of growth. Accurate reduction is important to reconstruct the joint surface.

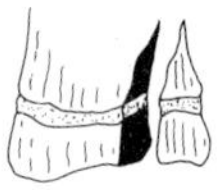

Type 4. Transepiphyseal fracture. Unless precisely realigned, union will occur between the epiphysis of one fragment and the metaphysis of the other causing premature fusion which results in angulation and deformity.

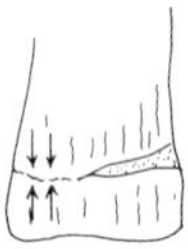

Type 5. This type is probably more common than is thought but it is not usually recognized until deformity occurs. There is a crush injury of the growth plate and diagnosis is difficult because there is rarely displacement. Premature fusion with deformity and shortening are inevitable.

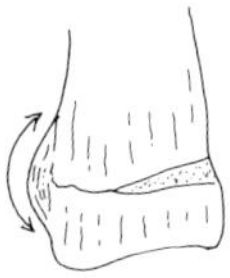

Type 6. A blow to the periosteum results in a bridge of bone being formed across the growth plate leading to angulation.

Fig. 90d

General principles for the treatment of fractures involving the growth plate

This section concerns the management of Salter Type 1 and 2 injuries where there is separation of the epiphysis, sometimes called epiphysiolysis.

1 Reduction of the epiphyseal separation should be carried out as early as possible—closed reduction is ideal

68

but it is often difficult to achieve owing to the small size of the epiphysis. If reduction is managed and the leg is immobilized in a cast, then minimal disturbance to longitudinal bone growth is likely.

2   In the majority of cases open reduction is necessary. This must be done with a minimum of trauma and great care should be taken to avoid leverage on the epiphyseal side of the growth plate, otherwise the germinal cells will be damaged and premature closure caused.

3   If internal fixation is used, the ideal method is Kirschner wires or small Steinman pins placed across the growth plate with as little deviation from the long axis of the bone as possible (Fig. 90e). Provided the pins do not occupy more than 20% of the surface area of the growth plate, then minimal disturbance in longitudinal growth will result. However, although the ideal method of fixation has been mentioned, the method will depend on the age of the animal and epiphysis involved. For example, when separation of the distal epiphysis of the femur has occurred in a puppy under 6 months of age, then crossed Kirschner wires (Fig. 90f) are the preferred method of fixation because they cause minimal interference with growth. However, they do not provide the stability of a screw. A screw (Fig. 90g) is used for fixation in larger dogs over 7 months of age because

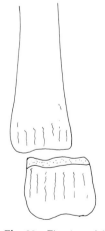

Fig. 90e. Fixation of the epiphysis in puppies under 6 months of age.

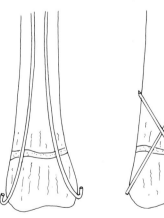

Fig. 90f. Fixation of the epiphysis in puppies under 6 months of age.

there is only limited growth potential left. The screw provides optimal stability and the fracture should heal with minimal callus formation, which is important as far as joint function is concerned. When screws are used to stabilize an epiphysis in puppies under 6 months of age, they must be removed after 3–4 weeks to prevent premature closure of the growth plate.

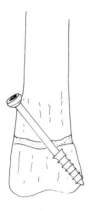

Fig. 90g. Screw fixation of epiphysis used in puppies over 7 months of age.

4   Epiphyseal separations and fractures heal very rapidly often within 4 weeks.

5   A puppy that has been treated for an epiphyseal separation or fracture must be checked at regular intervals in case shortening or angular deformity results. Often no matter how careful the reduction has been, premature closure of the growth plate occurs. If this results in loss in length of a bone, it is often of minor significance as dogs accommodate well to limb shortening. A far more serious complication is angular deformity and this is most commonly seen as a result of growth plate injuries of the radius and ulna (see page 172).

Shaft fractures in puppies

The management of fractures in puppies under 5 months of

age differs from methods described for adult dogs. Fractures heal very rapidly in 2–4 weeks. Plenty of callus is produced which undergoes rapid and complete remodelling, leaving none or very little evidence of the original fracture. Closed reduction and external fixation should be used whenever possible in puppies. However, Brinker, Piermattei and Flo (1983) recommend that internal fixation is indicated for:

1 Fractures causing rotational deformity or excessive shortening.
2 Displaced fractures of articular surfaces.
3 Fractures affecting the growth plate.

A small diameter intramedullary pin can be used for fixation of a shaft fracture because there is much more cancellous bone for the pin to embed in compared with the adult. Bone plates should rarely be used and are removed early (1 month).

Kirschner wires are used to reconstruct fractures involving joint surfaces—but in some cases a cancellous screw may be needed to give better stability.

REFERENCES

ALLGOWER M., MATTER P., PERREN S.M. & REUDI T. (1973) The dynamic compression plate (DCP). In: Springer Verlag, Berlin, Heidelberg, New York.

BRADEN T.D., BRINKER W.O., LITTLE R.W., JENKINS R.B. & BUTLER D. (1973) Comparative evaluations of bone healing in the dog. *J. Am. Vet. Med. Ass.* **163**, 65.

BRINKER W.O. PIERMATTEI D.L. & FLO G.L. (1983) *Handbook of Small Animal Orthopaedics and Fracture Treatment.* W.B. Saunders Company, Philadelphia, London. 195.

BRINKER W.O., FLO G.L. & LAMMERDINE J.J. *et al* (1977) Guidelines for selecting proper implant size for treatment of fractures in the dog and cat. *J. Am. Anim. Hosp. Ass.* **13**, 476.

COHEN J. & HARRIS W.H. (1958) The three dimensional anatomy of haversian systems. *J. Bone & Joint Surg.* **40A**, 419.

KUNTSCHER G. (1965) Intramedullary surgical technique and its place in orthopaedic surgery. *J. Bone & Joint Surg.* **47A**, 809.

MULLER M.E., ALLGOWER M. & WILLENEGGER H. (1970) *Manual of Internal Fixation,* Springer Verlag, Berlin, Heidelberg, New York.

NEWTON C.D. & HOHN R.B. (1974) Fracture non–union resulting from cerclage appliances. *J. Am. Vet. Med. Ass.* **164**, 503.

PAUWELS F. (1965) *Gesammelte Aghandlungen zur Funktionellen Anatomie les bewegungs-apparates.* Springer Verlag, Berlin, Heidelberg, New York.

Rush L. (1955) *Atlas of Rush Pin Techniques*. The Berivon Company, Meridian, Miss.

Salter R.B., & Harris W.R. (1963) Injuries involving the epiphyseal plate. *J. Bone Jt Surgery* **45A**, 587.

Vaughan L.C. (1975) Complications associated with the internal fixation of fractures in the dog. *J. small Anim. Pract.* **16**, 415.

Withrow S.J. & Homberg D.C. (1972) Use of full cerclage wires in the fixation of 18 consecutive long bone fractures in small animals. *J. Am. Anim. Hosp. Ass.* **13**, 735.

Chapter 3
The Skull and Spine

THE SKULL

Fractures of the mandible

The common sites of mandibular fracture are:
1   The symphysis.
2   The horizontal ramus between the canine and first premolar teeth.
3   The horizontal ramus at the level of the carnassial tooth.
4   The junction of the horizontal and vertical ramus.

The vertical ramus is less prone to fracture because it is well protected by muscle and the zygomatic arch.

The majority of mandibular fractures are caused in road traffic accidents. Kicks, bites, gun shot wounds and dentistry account for the remaining cases. Paradontal disease predisposes to fracture and could account for the relatively high incidence of the injury in Poodles and Pekingeses. Clinical signs of fracture include bleeding from the mouth, excessive salivation and malocclusion of the teeth. The jaw is displaced towards the side of fracture.

Although fractures of the mandible are usually compound, infection is seldom a serious problem due to the antibacterial and cleansing action of saliva (Weinmann and Sicher 1955). The aim of treatment is to immobilize the fracture and restore good occlusion of the teeth to allow an early return to normal feeding.

First aid immobilization of mandibular fractures is simply achieved by closing the mouth and applying a muzzle so that the upper jaw acts as a splint for the lower. A muzzle can be used as the sole method of treatment and is loosened at feeding times to allow the animal to drink liquids. The methods of fixation for mandibular fractures are listed below.

Fractures of the symphysis

Cerclage wire (Winstanley 1976)
Good fixation of the symphysis can be achieved with a cerclage wire placed around the mandible just caudal to the canine teeth (Fig. 91). The wire is passed under the soft tissues so that it lies in close contact with the bone. A large hypodermic needle is bent into a half circle; it can be used as a guide to pass the wire around the symphysis (Fig. 91). The

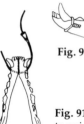

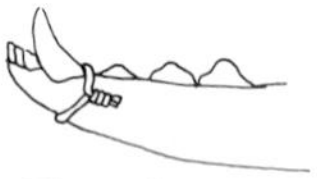

Fig. 91b

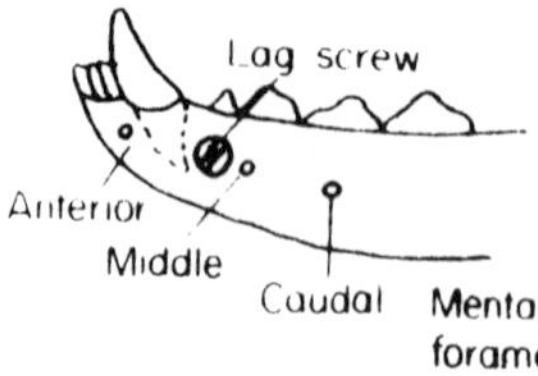

Lag screw

Anterior
Middle
Caudal   Mental
foramen   **Fig. 92**

Fig. 91a. Needle used
to guide wire
round symphysis.

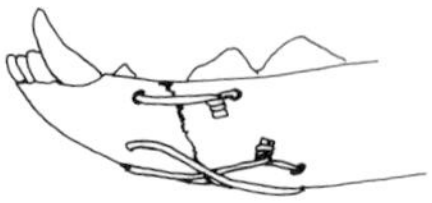

Fig. 93

cerclage wire tends to become buried beneath the mucous membrane and can be left *in situ*. The symphysis should heal within five weeks; if the wire is still visible or causing soft tissue reaction it is removed after this period.

The lag screw (Lawson 1963; Wolff 1974)
The mucous membrane is elevated and a lag screw inserted transversely just behind the canine teeth and anterior to the middle mental foramen (Fig. 92). This method provides optimal stability and avoids vital structures.

Transverse pin (Leonard 1971; Spellman 1972)
An alternative to the lag screw is to transfix the mandible with a pin (site of entry is as in Fig. 92).

FRACTURES OF THE HORIZONTAL RAMUS OF
THE MANDIBLE

Anterior ramus (Fig. 93)
A wire suture is placed close to the buccal margin of the

74

fracture. Holes for the wire are drilled between the teeth roots. Stability can be improved by placing a wire tension band over the ventral aspect of the fracture. Exposure is achieved through a ventral skin incision.

FRACTURES OF THE HORIZONTAL RAMUS CAUDAL TO THE SECOND PREMOLAR TOOTH

Plate Fixation (Sumner-Smith & Dingwall 1971, 1973)
Application of a plate to the lateral surface of the mandible close to the ventral border is the most satisfactory method of fixation for fractures of the horizontal ramus. It is essential that the plate is carefully contoured to the shape of the bone to prevent mal-occlusion. Exposure of the fracture is through a skin incision over the ventral aspect of the ramus. The platysma muscle is incised and retracted dorsally to expose the bone (Fig. 94).

Application of the plate close to the ventral border of the ramus (Fig. 95) avoids the risk of penetration of tooth roots and the mandibular nerve by screws.

Transverse pinning (Lawson 1957)
Transverse pinning is a simple and effective form of fixation. The pin passes horizontally posterior to the fracture through the sublingual tissue and must be inserted at right angles to the median plane through all cortices (Fig. 96).

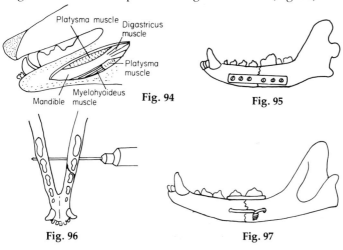

Platysma muscle Digastricus muscle
Platysma muscle
Myelohyoideus muscle
Mandible muscle
Fig. 94

Fig. 95

Fig. 96

Fig. 97

75

Wire sutures

Wire sutures placed around the base of teeth or through holes drilled in the bone can be used for fixation in small dogs (Fig. 97). Whatever fixation is used for fractures of the horizontal ramus of the mandible an attempt should be made to repair torn gums and buccal mucous membrane to limit further contamination of the fracture site.

FRACTURES OF THE VERTICAL RAMUS

The vertical ramus is well protected by muscle and provided there is little displacement of the fragments fractures of this region can be treated conservatively (Lawson 1963). However plate fixation has been described (Sumner Smith & Dingwall 1971). A skin incision is made over the angle of the jaw (Fig. 98). The periosteum is incised along the caudal aspect of the ramus and elevated with the attached masseter muscle to expose the vertical ramus taking care to avoid the vital structures shown in Fig. 99. Small ASIF plates are ideal for fracture fixation using 2.0 or 2.7 mm cortex screws.

FRACTURES OF THE MANDIBLE–AFTERCARE

Liquid or soft food should be fed for at least three weeks after fixation. Occasionally dogs with severe trauma to the jaw may need feeding through a pharyngostomy tube for a few days after surgery. Systemic antibiotics are indicated in all cases where the fracture is compound. If malocclusion prevents eating then extraction of the offending teeth may be necessary.

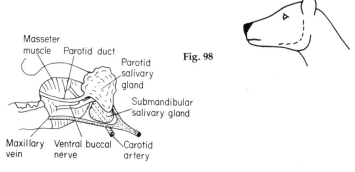

Fig. 98

Masseter muscle Parotid duct
Parotid salivary gland
Submandibular salivary gland
Maxillary vein Ventral buccal nerve Carotid artery

Fig. 99 reproduced by permission of Sumner-Smith G. & Dingwall J.S. (1973). The plating of mandibular fractures in the dog. *Vet. Rec.* **92,** 39.

Fractures of the nasal, premaxilla and maxillary bones

Although fractures of these bones are often initially associated with epistaxis and obstruction of the nasal passages this is usually a transient problem and the fractures will heal without surgical interference. Occasionally a dog will be encountered with gross instability of the nose resulting from multiple fractures. Under these circumstances fixation can be provided by half pin splintage. The fragments are transfixed with pins and the ends of the pins are incorporated in an acrylic resin 'bumper' moulded round the nose (Fig. 100a,b).

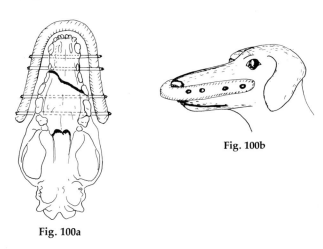

Fig. 100b

Fig. 100a

Fractures of the neurocranium
(Hoerlein 1971; Oliver 1975)

Fractures of the neurocranium may be associated with brain damage either directly or indirectly by haemorrhage into the cranial vault. Associated signs will of course vary with the degree or location of brain damage. Linear fractures require no treatment except rest provided there is no evidence of intracranial haemorrhage. However, cranial decompression should be considered as an emergency procedure if any of the following signs are present and progressive:
1 Loss of consciousness.

2   Dilation of one or both pupils or other evidence of cranial nerve injury.

3   Motor dysfunction such as hemiparesis or decerebrate rigidity.

Pressure may be relieved by trephining the skull close to the fracture.

Depression fractures may impinge on or lacerate the cerebral cortex. Pressure should be relieved as quickly as possible by careful elevation of the fragments from the dura mater, haemorrhage is controlled and the dura closed either by direct suture or by application of a temporal fascia graft if a defect is present. Closure of the dura mater is important because of its function as a barrier to infection of the central nervous system. The defect in the skull is covered with the temporal muscle. Alternatively if the fragment is large it may be retained in position with wire sutures.

Luxation of the temporomandibular joint
(Leonard 1971; Knecht & Schiller 1974)

Open 'jaw locking' as a result of temporomandibular luxation is a well-recognized but uncommon clinical entity in the dog. Traumatic over-extension of the temporomandibular joint results in forward and upward displacement of the mandibular condyle.

Under general anaesthesia manual reduction is achieved by placing a fulcrum (1–3 cm diameter wooden rod) transversely across the mouth. This procedure moves the man-

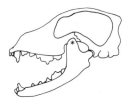

Fig. 101

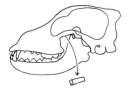

Fig. 102

Figs 101 and 102 reproduced by permission of Robins G.N. & Grandage J. (1977). Temporomandibular joint dysplasis and open mouth jaw locking in the dog. *J. Am. Med. Ass.* **171**, 1072.

dibular condyle backwards and ventrally to re-engage the temporal joint surface. It may be necessary to tape the mouth closed (between meals) for ten to fourteen days to maintain reduction.

Subluxation of the temporomandibular joint
(Cameron *et al* 1975; Robins & Grandage 1977)

Subluxation of the temporomandibular joint may result in repeated bouts of open mouth jaw locking. The condition is encountered in Basset Hounds and a single case has also been described in an Irish Setter. It has been suggested that the primary aetiological factor is temporomandibular dysplasia.

This allows the coronoid process* to become displaced lateral to the rostral part of the zygomatic arch as the mouth is closed and prevents closure (Fig. 101). The condition can be relieved by resection of the ventral part of the zygomatic arch (Fig. 102).

Mandibular neurapraxia (Robins 1976)

Mandibular neurapraxia is the term used to describe a condition in the dog which is probably caused by bilateral, temporary paralysis of the mandibular branch of the trigeminal nerve as a result of wide opening of the mouth.

In affected cases the lower jaw hangs down passively but manipulation of the mandible is not resented and the mouth can be passively closed. However, the lower jaw drops as soon as it is released. The condition usually resolves within three weeks. The mouth is kept loosely muzzled during this period and the dog is fed a semi-liquid diet with the muzzle in place.

Mandibular neurapraxia should be differentiated from other conditions which result in inability to close the mouth such as:
1   Oral foreign body.
2   Fracture of the mandible.
3   Luxation or subluxation of the temporomandibular joint.

Neurological examination (Palmer 1965; Griffiths 1972)

The basic layout of the central nervous system (CNS) is simply illustrated in Fig. 103. The system can be divided into two parts, the lower motor neurone and the upper motor neurone. The lower motor neurone is the effector unit of the CNS and consists of a ventral horn cell, its axon and termination in voluntary muscle. The upper motor neurone relays impulses from the cerebral cortex via the corticospinal tracts to the lower motor neurone (Fig. 103).

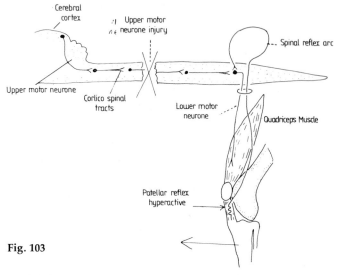

Fig. 103

The lower motor neurone is not only activated by the upper motor neurone but also by local reflex arcs. The activity of these reflex arcs is influenced and modified by the upper motor neurone. Hence injury to the spinal cord at the thoraco-lumbar junction tends to disrupt upper motor neurone control over the hind legs. Although reflex activity in the legs remains, it is hyperactive because the inhibitory effect of the upper motor neurones has been lost.

Lower motor neurone injury in clinical cases is usually synonymous with peripheral nerve injury so that both motor and sensory components are lost, the result is:

1   Loss of voluntary motor activity.

2   Loss of reflex motor activity.   4   Fibrillation.
3   Loss of tone and flaccidity.   5   Muscle atrophy.

Peripheral nerve injury—the forelimb

The brachial plexus is derived from the last three cervical and first two thoracic nerves. The nerves of the forelimb and the muscles they supply are given in Fig. 108. Worthman (1957) carried out experimental neurectomies in the dog and demonstrated that, with the exception of the radial nerve, nerves of the forelimb could be sectioned without producing an alteration in the dog's gait although the dependant muscles atrophied. Section of the radial nerve resulted in paralysis of the extensors of the elbow, carpus and digits. The limb was held in flexion and could bear no weight. There was desensitization of the dorsal and lateral parts of the forearm and dorsal aspect of the paw.

Worthman (1957) considers that the most common causes of radial nerve paralysis are fractures of the first rib and humerus. However, many dogs presented after road accidents with apparent radial nerve paralysis have an avulsion of the brachial plexus. In the most severely affected cases this injury results in paralysis of all forelimb muscle groups with accompanying sensory loss. Most cases of avulsion of the brachial plexus have a very poor prognosis for a useful recovery of limb function (Griffiths *et al* 1974). Amputation is indicated if there is no evidence of recovery within three months, or earlier, should the limb become severely excoriated by contact with the ground or by self-mutilation.

What are the alternatives to amputation?

Skin flap
A 'web' of skin may be established in the angle of the elbow

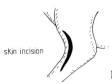

skin incision

Fig. 104

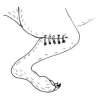

Fig. 105

81

to keep the joint in flexion and prevent excoriation of the lower limb by contact with the ground (Figs 104 and 105).

Carpal arthrodesis

In dogs with low lesions of the radial nerve that are able to extend the elbow but still knuckle at the carpus, fusion of the carpus may help to restore limb function. However, in the author's experience dogs treated in this way may continue to have problems due to knuckling of the digits with excoriation of the skin.

Muscle relocation techniques (Bennett & Vaughan, 1976)

Limb function can be restored or improved in dogs with certain peripheral nerve injuries by means of muscle relocation techniques. Successful application of this method is dependant on the availability of a muscle from a different group to the paralysed muscles, which must have an intact nerve supply and must be in a position to allow physical transposition. These criteria are difficult to fulfil as more than one nerve is often injured as in brachial plexus avulsion.

After radial nerve paralysis elbow function can be restored by cutting the tendon of insertion of the biceps brachii muscle and relocating the point of insertion to the posterior medial aspect of the olecranon where the tendon is sutured to the periosteum. Ability to extend the carpus and digits is restored by side-to-side anastomosis between the tendon of the flexor carpi radialis or flexor carpi ulnaris muscle and the common digital extensor tendon. After successful treatment an improvement in limb function should occur within 6 weeks with recovery in 3 months.

Hind limb peripheral nerve injury

The lumbosacral plexus is derived from the last three lumbar and the first three sacral nerves. The clinical signs associated with paralysis of specific nerves of the hind limb have been described by Worthman (1957).

OBTURATOR NERVE

This innervates the external obturator, pectineus, adductor

and gracilis muscle. Obturator paralysis therefore results in an inability to adduct the limb.

FEMORAL NERVE
This innervates the quadriceps muscle group and paralysis results in inability to protract or fix the stifle when weight bearing which in turn leads to collapse of the hock. Sensation is lost on the medial aspect of the leg.

SCIATIC NERVE
This innervates the hamstring muscle group and then terminates in the peroneal and the tibial nerves which supply all the muscles below the stifle. The peroneal innervates the extensors of the digits and flexors of the hock. Paralysis results in hyperextension of the hock and knuckling of the digits. Muscle relocation techniques have been used to restore limb function following peroneal nerve paralysis (Bennett & Vaughan, 1976). A side-to-side anastomosis is performed between the tendon of the functional long digital flexor and the tendon of the nonfunctional long digital extensor muscle.

Upper motor neurone lesions

Upper motor neurone lesions result in spastic paralysis in which there is
1   Limited voluntary movement.
2   Intact reflex activity which is often hyperactive.
3   Increased tone.
4   Abnormal reflexes—uncontrolled tail wag when a hind limb is stimulated, involuntary urination (mass reflex) in response to stimulation of the hindquarters.
   The commonest site of cord compression is in the thoracolumbar region most often as a result of a disc protrusion. Clinical signs can be divided into 5 groups according to the severity of cord compression.
1   Thoracolumbar pain.
2   Thoracolumbar pain and paresis of the hind limbs.
3   Paraplegia with local reflex activity and sensation present in the hind limbs.

4   Paraplegia with local reflex activity but no sensation present in the hind limbs.

5   Flaccid paralysis.

Paralysis of the hind limbs associated with disc protrusion in the thoraco lumbar region is usually spastic in nature unless there has been irreversible damage to the spinal cord with ascending and descending myelomalacia. In the neurological examination of the dog with hind limb paresis or paraplegia the withdrawal (pedal) reflex is assessed by pinching the interdigital skin of the foot. It is important to differentiate between a pedal reflex which can be present after complete cord transection and withdrawal of the limb due to pain, the latter is very important with regard to prognosis. When pinching the foot the dog's head end should be carefully observed for conscious reaction to pain.

The patellar reflex is tested by tapping the straight patellar ligament which should result in a reflex jerk of the limb. Muscle tone (resistance to passive movement) is best assessed by manipulation of the limb when the dog is lying on its side.

In the animal with hind leg ataxia conscious proprioception can be simply assessed by knuckling the foot. If the dog is aware that this has been done it will quickly return the foot to its normal position. An alternative is to stand the dog's foot on a piece of paper. The paper is moved away and if the dog is unaware of the position of its foot it will be moved passively on the paper.

The panniculus reflex is useful to assess the site of cord injury. Pricking or pinching the flank results in local contraction of the panniculus muscle. The muscle has a segmental sensory nerve supply from the first thoracic to the third lumbar nerve while its motor supply is derived from the lateral thoracic nerve. Reflex contraction is usually absent caudal to the site of cord injury.

Other signs or tests to indicate the site of cord compression are as follows:

1   Lesions cranial to the third lumbar vertebra disrupt the sypathetic nerve supply to the hind limbs resulting in hyperthermia through loss of vasomotor control.

2   Lesions between the third and fourth lumbar vertebrae result in a depressed patellar reflex.

3   Lesions between the fourth and sixth lumbar vertebrae result in hind leg weakness and urinary retention.

4   Lesions of the cauda equina are considered on page 115.

If there is radiographic evidence of cord compression in the thoracolumbar region (i.e. disc protrusion, fracture or dislocation) and the dog has flaccid paralysis of the hind legs, this usually indicates that there has been irreversible damage to the spinal cord with extensive haemorrhage and ascending myelomalacia. It is important to recognize the *ascending syndrome* because it carries a hopeless prognosis and affected animals should be destroyed on humane grounds. The clinical signs of the ascending syndrome are:

1   Generalized pain and dullness.

2   Flaccid paralysis of the hind legs, tail and anal sphincter.

3   Penis hangs flaccidly from the prepuce.

4   As myelomalacia extends cranially, the Schiff Sherrington reflex becomes apparent in which there is rigid extension of both forelegs.

5   Later the forelegs become flaccid.

6   Death occurs 5 or 6 days after the onset of paraplegia when there is involvement of the phrenic outflow at C5, C6 and C7.

Flaccid paralysis of the hind limbs can also be caused by a *spontaneous spinal haemorrhage*. The condition tends to be seen in young dogs of the larger breeds. It can be differentiated from the ascending syndrome in that there is often pain sensation still present in the hind legs, despite the paralysis. Radiographs of the spine are normal and approximately 65% of dogs recover the use of their hind legs within 6 weeks.

Conditions which should be considered in a differential diagnosis of hind leg paresis, ataxia or paraplegia are listed below.

Conditions causing a sudden onset of paraplegia include:

1   Thoracolumbar disc protrusion—commonest sites T12/13, T13/L1.

2   Spinal fractures and dislocations—commonest sites

terminal thoracic and terminal lumbar regions.

3   Spontaneous spinal haemorrhage.

4   Cord infarction caused by fibrocartilaginous embolism (De Lahunta & Alexander 1976; Hayes *et al* 1978).

Conditions causing a gradual onset of paresis or ataxia include:

1   Chronic Degenerative Radiculomyelopathy (CDRM) (Griffiths & Duncan 1975). This condition is seen in older dogs of the larger breeds, especially the German Shepherd. There is a slowly progressive ataxia and weakness of the hind legs. The nails tend to be excessively worn and there are deficits in conscious proprioception. The patellar reflex is often depressed. There are degenerative lesions in the lumbar dorsal columns and the condition has been classified as a 'dying back' disease of the central nervous system. Affected animals are usually destroyed 6 months to 1 year from the time of diagnosis because of the increasing severity of hind leg ataxia. There is no effective treatment. CDRM is sometimes confused with hip dysplasia. Admittedly, many older dogs presented with CDRM will have radiographic evidence of hip dysplasia and osteoarthritis but this is often of no clinical significance unless there is obvious pain on manipulation of the hips. Hip dysplasia does not cause deficits in conscious proprioception and excessive wear of the nails!

2   Cervical Spondylopathy (see page 91).

3   Giant Axonal neuropathy (Duncan & Griffiths 1981). Affects German Shepherds 14–15 months of age. Clinical signs include hind leg weakness and ataxia. Megaloesophagus appears to be a cardinal feature of the disease.

4   Distal Denervating Disease. (Griffiths & Duncan, 1979). A degenerative neuropathy of the distal motor axon in dogs. Affected animals present with quadriparesis, local reflex activity is depressed and there is muscle atrophy. Spontaneous recoveries have been recorded.

5   Progressive Axonopathy of Boxer dogs. (Griffiths, Duncan & Baker 1980). The disease is inherited as an autosomal recessive trait. The age of onset is usually between three and six months. The main presenting sign is an ataxia of the hind limbs, decreased muscle tone, absence

of the patellar reflexes, preservation of the pedal reflexes, good conscious pain sensation and virtual absence of muscle atrophy. The signs are symmetrical. Nerve roots and, to a lesser extent, peripheral nerves show demyelination/remyelination changes.

6   Demyelination of the cord due to distemper virus or toxoplasmosis.

7   Spinal tumours.

Clinical signs associated with lesions of the cervical spinal cord include:

1   Pain.

2   Pain and foreleg paresis.

3   Hemiparesis.

4   Quadriparesis.

5   Quadriplegia.

However in the condition cervical spondylopathy (Canine Wobbler syndrome), although the site of cord compression is in the cervical region hind leg ataxia is the main presenting sign.

The radiographic diagnosis of spinal lesions is dependant upon good positioning and a demonstration of fine detail. General anaesthesia is essential to allow correct positioning of the dog. Lateral views of the spine are usually the most helpful but should be supplemented by ventrodorsal views as necessary. The long axis of the spine does not normally lie parallel to the table top when the dog is lying on its side, so soft pads must usually be placed under the nose, neck and lumbar spine (Fig. 106).

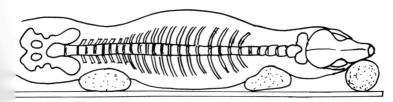

Fig. 106

The sagittal plane through the vertebrae should also be parallel to the film. This is achieved by keeping the upper legs parallel to the top of the table with pads (Fig. 107).

The neurological examination of the spine and peripheral nerves is summarized in Fig. 108.

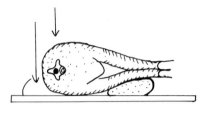

Fig. 107

CERVICAL SPINE

Atlanto-axial subluxation (Geary *et al* 1967; Gage & Smallwood 1970; Ladds *et al* 1970; Gage 1975)

Atlanto-axial subluxation is occasionally encountered in toy breeds of dogs particularly Pomeranians and Yorkshire terriers. The condition is characterized by compression of the cervical spinal cord with pain and motor dysfunction. Clinical signs usually become apparent before the dog reaches a year of age. Four specific anatomical abnormalities may result in atlanto-axial subluxation. These include:

1   Congenital absence of the dens which is said to be the most common.
2   Congenital odontoid process separation.
3   Tearing or stretching of the ligaments between the atlas and axis.
4   Fracture of the odontoid process with concurrent rupture of the atlanto-axial ligament.

Onset of clinical signs may be sudden or gradual, the former being the most common. The signs include cervical pain and motor dysfunction ranging from paresis of the fore or hind legs to total quadriplegia.

A lateral radiograph of the cervical spine with the head in a flexed position will confirm the presence of atlanto-axial subluxation (Figs 109 and 110).

The luxation can be reduced and the vertebrae stabilized by a wire suture (24 gauge) passed under the dorsal

88

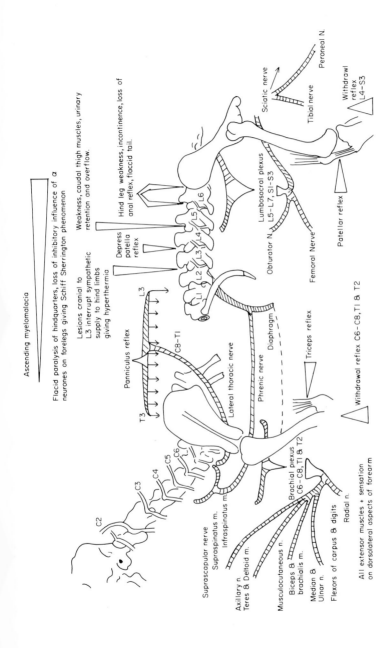

Ascending myelomalacia

Flacid paralysis of hindquarters, loss of inhibitory influence of α neurones on forelegs giving Schiff Sherrington phenomenon

Lesions cranial to L3 interrupt sympathetic supply to hind limbs giving hyperthermia

Weakness, caudal thigh muscles, urinary retention and overflow.

Hind leg weakness, incontinence, loss of anal reflex, flaccid tail.

Depress patella reflex

Panniculus reflex

L3

C8–T1

T3

Lateral thoracic nerve

Phrenic nerve

Diaphragm

Triceps reflex

Withdrawal reflex C6–C8, T1 & T2

Brachial plexus C6–C8, T1 & T2

Suprascapular nerve
Supraspinatus m.
Infraspinatus m.

Axillary n.
Teres & Deltoid m.

Musculocutaneous n.
Biceps & brachialis m.

Median & Ulnar n.

Flexors of corpus & digits

Radial n.

All extensor muscles + sensation on dorsolateral aspects of forearm

Lumbosacral plexus L5–L7, S1–S3

Obturator N. L3–L7

Femoral Nerve

Patellar reflex

Sciatic nerve

Tibial nerve

Peroneal N.

Withdrawl reflex L4–S3

C2
C3
C4
C5
C6

L1 L2 L3 L4 L5 L6

Fig. 108. Neurological examination—summary.

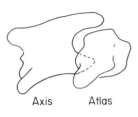

Fig. 109. Normal alignment of the atlas and axis.

Axis   Atlas

Subluxation

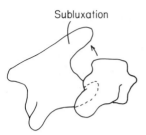

Fig. 110. Dorsal tilting of the spine of the axis is seen in the subluxation.

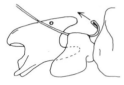

Fig. 111

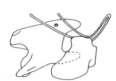

Fig. 112

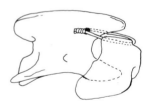

Fig. 113

arch of the atlas and through the dorsal spine of the axis (Figs 111, 112 and 113). A dorsal midline approach is used to expose the vertebrae.

In addition a cancellous bone graft may be packed around the wire sutures to promote bony union between the vertebrae as the wires alone may break with time with a recurrence of symptoms.

Manipulation during surgery may result in respiratory arrest. Respiratory failure may also occur post-operatively due to oedema of the cord. Consequently the animal should be carefully monitored during anaesthesia and for 24 hours post-operatively. Steroids are given to control oedema. Antibiotic cover is also provided.

Cervical pain should abate within a few days of surgery and motor dysfunction resolve within 4–8 weeks. This is dependent on the time lapse between onset of signs and treatment and also the degree of damage to the cord.

Cervical spondylopathy (Canine Wobbler Syndrome)

Denny *et al* (1977) described 35 cases of cervical spondylopathy in the dog. The reader is referred to this paper (and to work by Read *et al* 1983), for the relevant literature review. Cervical spondylopathy is a syndrome characterized by a hind leg ataxia which is now recognized in certain breeds of dogs, notably the Great Dane and the Doberman Pinscher. The pathogenesis of the syndrome is not completely understood but is currently ascribed to compression of the cervical spinal cord, either as a result of instability of one or more of the vertebrae (Fig. 114) or as a result of deformity of a vertebra usually C6 or C7 causing stenosis of the canal (Fig. 115). Alternatively, both instability and deformity may coexist.

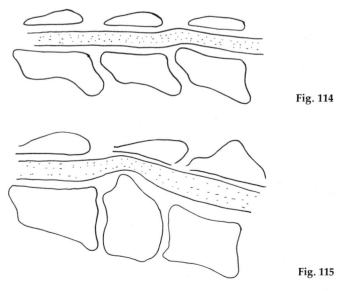

Fig. 114

Fig. 115

The condition appears to be most prevalent in the Great Dane and the Doberman Pinscher but it also has been recognized in the following breeds:

Basset Hound	Chow
St Bernard	Pyrenean Mountain Dog
Rhodesian Ridgeback	Retriever
Old English Sheepdog	Irish Setter
Boxer	English Mastiff
German Pointer	Borzoi
Rough Collie	English Pointer
Weimaraner	

In Great Danes male animals are usually affected while the sex distribution in other breeds is equal. 70% of Danes are under 1 year of age at the onset of clinical signs. Only 30% of Dobermans are under a year of age, the rest present between 1 and 12 with a peak at 4 years.

Animals are presented with variable histories which include clumsiness, difficulty in rising from a prone position, hind leg weakness, falling or collapse at exercise, cervical pain and, in the case of male dogs, inability to cock the leg or serve bitches.

Affected animals have hind leg ataxia and there is also forelimb involvement in some. Ataxia is most obvious at the walk and can be exacerbated by making the animal turn sharply. In extreme cases this manoeuvre results in loss of balance and collapse, while in others it induces crossing or wide abduction of the hind limbs. Some dogs resume an almost normal action when made to run a straight course. The main finding on neurological examination is a deficit in conscious proprioception. Knuckling of the digits, with excessive wear of the nails is a common finding. Cervical pain may be present and passive flexion of the neck can result in transient collapse.

Radiographic examination is necessary to confirm the clinical diagnosis of cervical spondylopathy. The examination is carried out under general anaesthesia with the animal in lateral recumbency. Radiographs of severely affected cases show evidence of gross misalignment of adjacent vertebrae or deformity, with the neck positioned conventionally in extension (Figs 114 and 115). More commonly, however, particularly in younger animals, flexed radiographs are required to demonstrate conclusively the characteristic upward tilting of the anterior borders of affected vertebral bodies.

In order to obtain full flexion of each cervical vertebral segment it is necessary to flex the entire spinal column so that the animal lies in a curled up position. Careful padding of the lower neck is required in order to avoid sagging which causes overlapping of the interspaces by obliquely projected vertebral end-plates. The muzzle is also raised, so that the sagittal plane of the skull is parallel to the table top. This position should be maintained for as short a time as possible since it tends to produce respiratory airway obstruction. A survey at this clinic suggests that cervical spondylopathy is a widespread problem in the Doberman Pinscher. Forty clinically normal dogs belonging to breeders were screened radiographically and vertebral instability was confirmed in every case. Approximately 30% of Dobermans have evidence of cervical disc protrusion. This has probably occurred secondary to vertebral instability and accounts for the sudden onset of clinical signs in some older dogs.

On confirmation of the diagnosis, owners should be advised that the ataxia is likely to become progressively worse and may be further complicated by urinary and faecal incontinence. However, progression may be arrested or resolved after surgical treatment. Most owners who opt for conservative treatment which simply involves restricted exercise usually request euthanasia within six months because of the progressively worsening ataxia. Surgical treatment should only be recommended for mature dogs in which cervical instability alone is demonstrated as the cause of cord compression. 50% of cases make complete recoveries and a further 20% improve following cervical fusion.

When stenosis exists it is possible to relieve cord compression by laminectomy (removal of the neural arch) but although the dog's action may improve following this procedure ataxia tends to recur as the neural arch reforms (Sumner Smith 1974; personal communication).

Cervical fusion is achieved by screw fixation of the vertebral bodies using the technique described by Gage & Hoerlein (1975). A ventral midline approach is used (see cervical disc fenestration, page 99). The vertebrae to be stabilized are exposed by cutting the attachments of the longus colli muscle to the ventral process, the muscle is then elevated from the vertebral body and retained laterally with retractors. A large window is cut in the ventral surface of the intervertebral disc and the nucleus pulposus removed with a dental tartar scraper (Fig. 116).

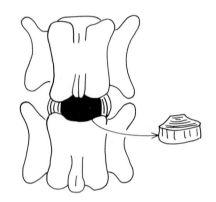

Fig. 116

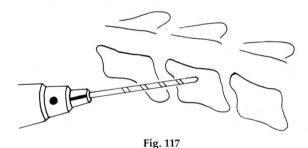

Fig. 117

The drill hole for each screw is started in the ventral midline at approximately the caudal third of the cranial vertebra. The drill bit is carefully advanced in a caudodorsal direction across the intervertebral space to end in the middle of the caudal vertebral body (Fig. 117).

A large bit is used to overdrill the hole in the cranial

94

vertebral body so that when the screw is inserted the two vertebrae will be lagged together. A depth gauge is inserted into the hole and advanced until its tip meets the cortex forming the roof of the caudal vertebral body. A screw is selected which is about 4 mm shorter than the length indicated by the gauge in order to avoid the risk of the screw point entering the spinal canal as it is tightened. A single screw is placed through the cranial and caudal part of the body of each unstable vertebra to ensure optimal stability (Fig. 118). As many as five consecutive vertebrae have been fused without apparent interference with the range of neck movement.

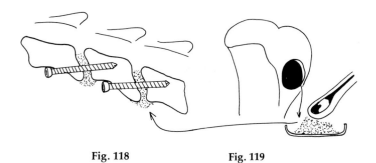

Fig. 118   Fig. 119

A graft of cancellous bone is obtained from the proximal humerus (Fig. 119) and packed around the invertebral disc spaces to promote early bony fusion. Routine wound closure is then undertaken. Radiographs are taken post-operatively to check the position of the screw. It is not always possible to restore normal alignment of the vertebrae but this does not seem to interfere with recovery provided complete stability is restored. Exercise should be severely restricted for 4 weeks after surgery and a normal action should be resumed within 2 months. In some dogs changes in the cord appear to be irreversible there being no improvement or deterioration in the degree of ataxia following cervical fusion.

What are the possible causes of cervical spondylopathy?

Diet
The nutritional status of affected animals is invariably normal.

Mechanical factors
It has been suggested that a large head on a long neck may impose abnormal stress on growing vertebrae. This might apply to the Great Dane but not the Doberman Pinscher.

Trauma
An injury can precipitate clinical signs, particularly in the older dog.

GENETIC FACTORS
Evidence that cervical spondylopathy is an inherited defect is provided by:
1   The disproportionate breed incidence in Dobermans and Great Danes.
2   The occurrence of the disorder in littermates.
3   The sex incidence in the Great Dane, the majority of animals being male.

As cervical spondylopathy appears to be so widespread in the Doberman, eradication by planned breeding seems impracticable. However, it is obviously unwise to continue to breed from animals which are known to have produced offspring with clinical signs of cervical spondylopathy.

Cervical disc protrusion

The normal intervertebral disc consists of the outer annulus fibrosus and the inner nucleus pulposus (Fig. 120).

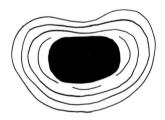

Fig. 120

The nucleus pulposus is a gel-like structure which develops from the notochord. The annulus fibrosus has an inner zone consisting of fibro-cartilage and an outer zone of collagen lamellae. The nucleus pulposus is situated eccentrically within the annulus, the ventral annulus being one and a half times thicker than the dorsal. Consequently, most disc protrusions occur dorsally.

Hansen (1952) described disc degeneration and protrusion. He divided dogs into two groups, chondrodystrophoid and non-chondrodystrophoid breeds.

In the chondrodystrophoid breeds such as Dachshund and the Pekingese, the nucleus pulposus undergoes chondroid metamorphosis so that the nucleus is gradually replaced by hyaline cartilage. The process occurs between 8 months and 2 years of age.

In non-chondrodystrophoid dogs fibroid metamorphosis occurs with gradual replacement of the nucleus pulposus by collagenous tissue. This process occurs later in life usually between 8 and 10 years.

These changes in the character of the nucleus pulposus precede degeneration. The chondroid nucleus undergoes calcification and similar changes can occur in the fibroid nucleus although far less commonly. Concurrent changes occur in the annulus fibrosus with fragmentation of the collagen lamellae.

Disc protrusion can consist of a total rupture of the dorsal annulus fibrosus with loss of varying amounts of degenerative nucleus pulposus into the epidural space. Alternatively, there may be only partial rupture of the annulus fibrosus with dorsal bulging of the disc.

The clinical, radiological and pathological findings associated with cervical disc protrusion were described by Olsson & Hansen 1952. The same authors also described the technique of ventral fenestration of the affected disc. Since then several reports have been published on the management of dogs with cervical disc protrusion, these have been reviewed and the results of surgical treatment of a further 40 cases described (Denny 1978). The results of this paper are published here.

The condition is most commonly encountered in the Beagle, Jack Russell Terrier, Dachshund and Cocker Spaniel. Age at the onset of clinical signs ranges from 1 to 12 years, with a peak incidence at 5 and 8 years. The most common presenting sign is cervical pain. The pain is often intense and the animal will scream if touched or moved (there is a saying that a cervical protrusion can be diagnosed without seeing the dog because of the cries of pain as the animal is brought into the waiting room). In less marked cases, the only evidence of pain is tautness of the cervical muscles as the dog guards its neck against passive manipulation. Affected animals are miserable and apprehensive. A hunched up attitude is adopted, usually with the head held down. One of the first presenting signs noticed is difficulty or unwillingness to lower the head to eat or drink. In addition there may be neurological deficits ranging from unilateral foreleg paresis, which is the most common, to hemi-paresis, quadriparesis or quadriplegia.

Diagnosis of a cervical disc protrusion is confirmed by lateral radiograph of the cervical spine (Fig. 121). A narrow intervertebral disc space is taken as evidence of protrusion. Calcification of the disc is not necessarily of any clinical significance unless there is dorsal extrusion of calcified material into the neural canal.

The most common site of disc protrusion is between C2/C3 and dogs presented with cervical pain alone, often have protrusions of one of the first three cervical discs. Dogs presented with cervical pain associated with foreleg paresis, hemi-paresis or quadriplegia are more likely to have protrusion of one of the last 3 cervical discs. The management of cases with cervical disc protrusion can be conservative or surgical. However, recurrence is more likely when conservative methods are used. This was demonstrated by Russell & Griffiths (1968) in an analysis of 110 cases. They found that recurrence in conservatively treated dogs over a 3-year period was 36.3%, whereas it was only 5.6% in dogs treated by ventral fenestration. Conservative treatment involves cage rest for 3 weeks and analgesics are given to control pain. If cervical pain persists, or neurological deficits become apparent, then fenestration should be recommended. In the majority of cases, fenestration is the treatment of choice. The operation simply involves cutting a window in the ventral surface of the annulus fibrosus of the disc to allow the nucleus pulposus to be removed and the protrusion to subside (Fig. 127).

98

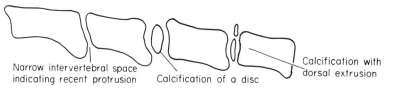

Narrow intervertebral space
indicating recent protrusion

Calcification of a disc

Calcification with
dorsal extrusion

Fig. 121. Radiographic changes in intervertebral disc disease.

If there has been complete rupture of the dorsal annulus fibrosus, then further extrusion of nucleus into the neural canal is prevented. The nucleus pulposus is replaced by scar tissue and therefore with regard to prophylaxis there is nothing further to be protruded or extruded into the neural canal.

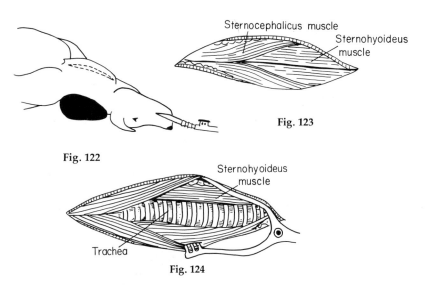

Sternocephalicus muscle

Sternohyoideus muscle

Fig. 123

Fig. 122

Sternohyoideus muscle

Trachea

Fig. 124

Cervical disc fenestration

The dog is placed in dorsal recumbency with the head extended over a sandbag and the forelimbs pulled back lateral to the chest (Fig. 122). A ventral midline skin incision is made extending from the level of the atlas to the manubrium sternum (Fig. 122). The paired bellies of the sternohyoideus muscles are divided along the midline and retracted to expose the trachea (Figs 123 and 124).

99

The trachea and oesophagus are retracted towards the left side of the neck and the right vagus and carotid artery displaced to the right to expose the longus colli muscle (Fig. 125). The position of a specific disc can be determined by first palpating the caudal border of the wings of the atlas and the ventral process of each vertebra caudal to this point. The intervertebral disc lies immediately caudal to the ventral process.

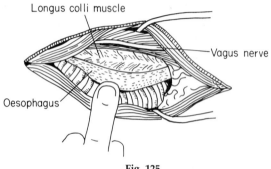

Fig. 125

The attachment of the longus colli muscle on each ventral process is cut. Self-retaining retractors are then used to displace the muscle laterally and expose the disc. A window is cut in the ventral surface of the intervertebral disc and the nucleus pulposus removed with a dental tartar scraper (Figs 126 and 127). The first 5 cervical discs are routinely fenestrated.

The defects in the longus colli muscle are sutured to prevent haemorrhage. The remaining muscle layers are coapted with a continuous suture of catgut and the skin with interrupted sutures.

Although fenestration provides effective relief from recurrence of cervical pain, 30% of dogs continue to have intermittent periods of pain for an average period of 2 weeks after surgery (Range 1–4 weeks). Severe neurological deficits as a result of disc protrusion are usually more commonly encountered in the thoracolumbar region as there is relatively little room for anything but the spinal cord within the neural canal. By comparison, the cervical neural canal is much larger than the cord, consequently disc protrusions in this region usually result in impingement on the nerve roots, causing pain and sometimes paresis of one limb rather than severe cord compression.

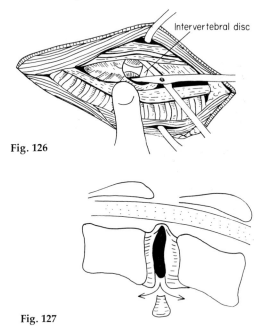

Fig. 126

Fig. 127

It may be argued that because of the relatively large space within the cervical neural canal that decompressive laminectomy is rarely necessary in dogs with cervical disc protrusion. The results of treatment by fenestration alone are encouraging in this respect. In dogs with cervical pain and foreleg paresis, paresis resolves within an average time of 3 weeks. In dogs with quadriparesis, the recovery period varies from 3–6 weeks. 50% of dogs with quadriplegia will recover provided fenestration is performed within 48 hours of the onset of signs.

THORACOLUMBAR SPINE

Thoracolumbar disc protrusions

Virtually all disc protrusions in the thoracolumbar region

occur between T11 and L4, the commonest site of protrusion being between T12/T13 and T13/L1.

The condition is most frequently encountered in the Dachshund and Pekingese. The clinical and radiological findings associated with protrusion have already been described (pages 83–85, 98).

Treatment of thoracolumbar disc protrusions may be conservative or surgical and Bojrab (1971) reported that the overall recovery rate was 85% based on the various methods of treatment reported in the literature. Conservative treatment involves enforced rest, preferably in a cage for 3/4 weeks. This type of treatment is recommended for the dog which has suffered its first attack of thoracolumbar pain or pain with hind leg paresis. Such dogs usually have dorsal protrusion of the disc without complete rupture of the annulus. Administration of corticosteroids or analgesics should be avoided in these cases. Otherwise pain relief with increased activity may result in a progression of the protrusion to rupture of the annulus with extrusion of the nucleus pulposus and severe cord compression. The paraplegic dog whether treated surgically or conservatively requires careful nursing. If urinary retention and overflow is present, the bladder should be expressed or drained by catheter at least twice daily. Antibiotic cover should be given to prevent urinary tract infection. Inability to move with urinary or faecal incontinence results in soiling of the coat and skin sores unless frequent bathing is carried out. The paraplegic dog must also be turned several times a day and bony prominences massaged to prevent the development of bed sores. Corticosteroids are given at high doses for 72 hours after the onset of paraplegia to reduce cord oedema.

Even when dogs recover after conservative treatment for a disc protrusion, there is a risk of recurrence and this risk can be minimized by surgical treatment.

A lateral approach for fenestration of thoracolumbar disc protrusions has been described by several authors (Seemann 1968, 1980; Flo & Brinker 1975; Denny 1978, 1983). Cases suitable for fenestration can be divided into four clinical categories:

1 Dogs with intractable or recurrent thoracolumbar pain. Fenestration usually provides rapid relief.

2 Dogs with hind leg paresis, with or without thoracolumbar pain and showing no response to conservative treatment within 3 weeks. The average recovery after fenestration is 4 weeks (range 2–8 weeks).

3 Paraplegic dogs with sensation in both hind legs with or without limited voluntary movement. Typically dogs in this group can almost stand when assisted, but drag their hind legs when made to walk. If the onset of paraplegia is sudden, fenestration should be performed within 3 days. Hind limb function is usually regained within 5 weeks (range 2–12 weeks). If the onset of paraplegia is gradual, surgery should be carried out within 8 days and the average recovery time is 5 weeks (range 2–12 weeks).

4 Paraplegic dogs with no sensation or voluntary movement in the hind limbs but pedal and patella reflexes present. The timing of surgery is critical for dogs in this category. If the onset of paraplegia is sudden, fenestration must be performed within 24 hours. Recovery periods range from 4 weeks to 4 months (average 9 weeks). If the onset is gradual (24 hours +), fenestration should be performed within a week and hind limb function is regained within an average time of 5.5 weeks (range 3–8 weeks).

The overall recovery rate for dogs in these categories is 91%, based on a series of 140 dogs treated at this clinic by fenestration of the last 3 thoracic and first 3 lumbar discs.

Surgical technique

Thoracolumbar disc fenestration is not an easy operation and initial practice on cadavers is recommended. Specialist instruments for the operation include 2 pairs of self–retaining retractors, dental tartar scrapers and a periosteal elevator. Suction is useful but not essential.

The dog is placed on its right side with the thoracolumbar region arched over a wooden pole (Fig. 128). (This widens the disc space laterally and makes fenestration easier; the pole is moved as necessary to improve exposure of individual discs). A lateral skin incision is made at the level of the transverse processes of the lumbar vertebrae from the ninth or tenth rib to the fifth lumbar vertebrae (Fig. 128). The subcutaneous fat is retracted to reveal the lumbo–dorsal

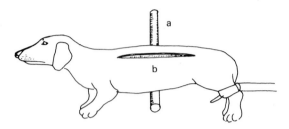

Fig. 128. The dog is placed on its right side with the thoracolumbar spine arched over a wooden pole (*a*). A lateral skin incision (*b*) is made from the ninth rib to the fifth lumbar vertebra.

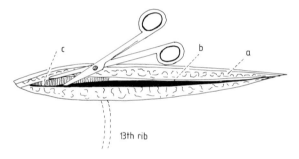

Fig. 129a. The subcutaneous fat (*a*), lumbodorsal fascia (*b*) and the latissimus dorsi muscle (*c*) are incised.

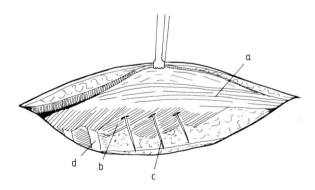

Fig. 129b. The lumbodorsal fascia and the latissimus dorsi muscle are retracted to reveal the longissimus dorsi (*a*) and the iliocostalis lumborum (*b*) muscles. The dorsal branches of the lumbar nerves (*c*) and the last two ribs (*d*) can also be seen.

104

fascia which merges with the latissimus dorsi muscle in the costal region. The fascia, muscle and underlying layer of fat are incised and retracted (Figs 129a and 129b). The longissimus dorsi and the iliocostalis lumborum muscles can then be identified (Fig. 129c). Although the two muscles are fused in the lumbar region they can be distinguished as the longissimus dorsi muscle, which lies dorsally, has a glistening silvery appearance, while the iliocostalis lumborum muscle presents fleshy serrations which insert on the transverse processes of the lumbar vertebrae and last four ribs. The iliocostalis lumborum muscle is detached and elevated from the last 3 ribs, and this area is packed with a swab to control haemorrhage (Fig. 129d) while the lumbar discs are being fenestrated.

Exposure of each of the first three lumbar discs is achieved by splitting the iliocostalis lumborum muscle in

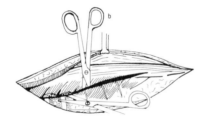

Fig. 129c. The iliocostalis lumborum muscle is detached and elevated from the last three ribs (*a*). The iliocostalis lumborum muscle is then split longitudinally over the first four lumbar transverse processes (*b*).

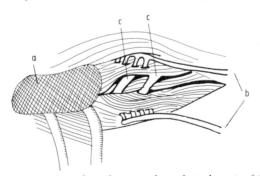

Fig. 129d. Haemorrhage from the severed costal attachments of the iliocostalis lumborum muscle is controlled by packing the area with a swab (*a*). Self-retaining retractors (*b*) are used to retract the iliocostalis lumborum muscle in the lumbar region while the transverse processes (*c*) are being exposed.

105

the direction of its fibres in a caudal direction from the transverse process of the second lumbar vertebra (Fig. 129c). The muscle is elevated from the transverse process of the second lumbar vertebra and exposure of the process maintained with self–retaining retractors (Fig. 129d). The first lumbar disc, covered by a layer of fascia, lies just cranial to the transverse process. Exposure is completed by elevation of fascia and muscle from the edge of the transverse process in a cranial direction. This is done initially with a periosteal elevator and the lateral surface of the disc is then cleaned with the corner of a dry swab held with artery forceps. Care is taken to avoid the ventral branch of the first lumbar nerve and its associated blood vessels which cross

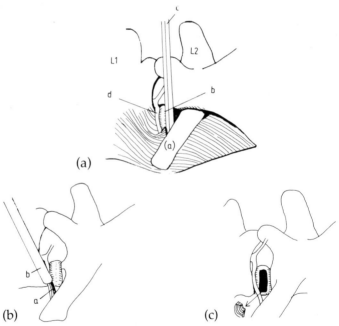

(a)

(b) (c)

Fig. 130a. The transverse process (*a*) of the second lumbar vertebra is cleared of muscle. The first lumbar disc (*b*) lies immediately cranial to the transverse process. Fascia covering the lateral aspect of the disc is cleared in a cranial direction using a periosteal elevator (*c*) initially. The ventral branch of the first lumbar nerve (*d*) crosses the cranial edge of the disc.

Fig. 130b. A vein (*a*) which runs with the spinal nerve is sometimes accidentally ruptured. Haemorrhage can be controlled by applying pressure with an elevator (*b*) on the tranioventral corner of the disc.

Fig. 130c. A window is cut through the lateral side of the annulus fibrosus and the nucleus pulposus is removed with a dental tartar scraper (*a*).

106

the craniolateral surface of the disc (Figs 130a,b). The vein is sometimes accidentally ruptured during exposure of the disc, but haemorrhage can be controlled by applying pressure with an elevator on the cranioventral corner of the disc (Fig. 130b). A 'window' is cut through the annulus fibrosus on the lateral side of the disc using a No. 15 scalpel blade and the nucleus pulposus is removed with a dental tartar scraper (Fig. 130c). The second and third lumbar and the thirteenth thoracic disc are exposed and fenestrated in the same way.

The swab covering the heads of the last 3 ribs is removed and exposure of the eleventh and twelfth thoracic discs carried out. These discs are covered by the levatores costorum muscles. Each muscle originates on the transverse process of a thoracic vertebra and inserts on the rib caudal to the process (Fig. 131). The origin of each muscle is partially severed with scissors (Fig. 131) and a periosteal elevator is used to retract the muscle in a ventral direction to complete exposure of the disc (Fig. 132). (Care is taken to avoid penetration of the pleural cavity during this procedure.)

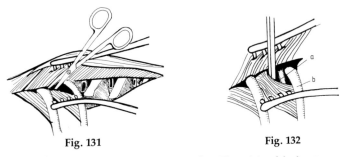

Fig. 131   Fig. 132

Fig. 131. Exposure of the twelfth thoracic disc. The origin of the levatores costorum muscle (a) is partially severed.

Fig. 132. Exposure of the twelfth thoracic disc. The levatores costorum muscle is retracted in a ventral direction to reveal the disc (a) lying just cranial to the head of the rib (b).

Lateral fenestration of the twelfth thoracic disc is then performed. Exposure and fenestration of the eleventh thoracic disc is achieved in the same way. Wound closure consists of separate layers of continuous 00 (BP) chromic catgut in the iliocostalis lumborum muscle, the latissimus dorsi fascia and the subcutaneous fat. The skin is coapted with simple interrupted or vertical mattress sutures of 00 monofilament nylon.

Post–operatively, antibiotic cover is given for 5 days and most dogs can be discharged within this period. Skin sutures are removed at 10 days and owners are given general advice on nursing the dog.

Dogs presented within 24 hours of a sudden onset of paraplegia are given high doses of hydrocortisone for 72 hours to control cord oedema. Dogs with urinary retention and overflow have their bladders emptied at least twice daily by catheter or manual expression until reflex emptying occurs (usually within 5 days). A frequent minor post–operative complication is flaccidity and bulging of the left abdominal wall. This is due to bruising of the ventral lumbar nerve roots during surgery. The flaccidity is a transient problem and normal muscle tone is regained within 2 weeks.

Dogs with severe hind leg paresis or paraplegia can also be treated by dorsal decompressive laminectomy (Funk-quist 1962) or by laminectomy and dorsolateral fenestration (Hoerlein 1956, 1971). However, paraplegic dogs with no sensation and only local reflex activity present in the hind limbs will recover after fenestration alone which brings the necessity of decompressive laminectomy into question (Flo & Bringer 1975; Denny 1978).

Spinal fractures and luxations

The most frequent site of spinal fracture in the dog is in the terminal thoracic region (Hoerlein 1971). In the cervical region fractures usually involve one of the first two cervical vertebrae while in the lumbar spine one of the last three vertebrae is most often affected.

FRACTURES OF THE CERVICAL VERTEBRAE
Fractures of the cervical vertebrae are uncommon in the dog (Stone *et al* 1979; Denny 1983). Fractures most often involve the atlas and axis. The commonest site axial fracture is the

dens and/or vertebral body.

Although there may be considerable displacement of fractures of the cranial cervical vertebrae, the resultant neurological deficits are often remarkably mild and the main presenting sign is cervical pain (De Lahunta 1977). However, deaths may occur from respiratory arrest when haemorrhage and oedema involve the brain stem following fracture (Gage 1968). Fractures of the caudal cervical vertebrae may cause quadriparesis or quadriplegia, and death may occur from respiratory failure if there is involvement of the phrenic outflow (De Lahunta 1977).

When fracture of a cervical vertebra is suspected, the dog must be handled with care to prevent further displacement of the fracture. Initial radiographic examination should ideally be carried out on the conscious animal. If the dog is anaesthetized for further radiographs or surgery then protective muscle tone is lost and the risk of fracture displacement is increased. This risk can be minimized by supporting the neck throughout the procedure and avoiding excessive flexion and extension. Diagnosis of cervical fracture can usually be confirmed from a lateral radiograph of the neck but in some cases ventrodorsal and oblique views may be necessary.

Most reported cases of cervical fracture have been treated surgically. Atlantoaxial subluxations with or without fractures of the dens have been stabilized by wiring the arch of the atlas to the dorsal spinous process of the axis (Figs 111–113, (Gage, 1968; Oliver & Lewis, 1973; Stone *et al* 1979)). When fractures have involved a cervical vertebral body, ventral plate fixation has been used (Stone *et al.* 1979) but experimental work by Swaim (1975) suggests that this technique is not always satisfactory as loosening of the screws and plate is a frequent complication. Another method of stabilizing cervical body fractures was described by Rouse (1979) with reference to three cases. Four pins were driven into the vertebral body, two cranial and two caudal to the fracture and were left protruding about 1 cm below the ventral aspect of the vertebral body. The fracture was reduced and the free ends of the pins were incorporated in bone cement which acted as an internal splint

(Fig. 133a). Rouse (1979), stresses the importance of reducing the fracture with the least possible trauma. Haemorrhage from the ventral vertebral sinus often occurs upon movement of the vertebral body fragments, and respiratory arrest is not uncommon, especially if extensive haemorrhage occurs within the neural canal. At this clinic nine dogs have been seen with fractures of the cervical vertebrae during a ten year period. The fractures involved the atlas in four dogs, the axis in four and the fifth cervical vertebra in one. Clinical signs included neck pain, quadriparesis or quadriplegia.

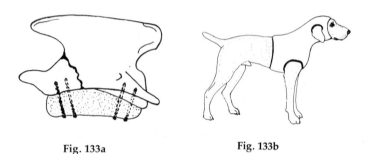

Fig. 133a   Fig. 133b

One dog in the series was treated surgically, the remainder were managed conservatively. Dogs with undisplaced cervical fractures were given strict rest for 4 weeks and those with displaced or unstable fractures had the neck immobilized in a plaster of Paris collar for 4 weeks (Fig. 133b). The cast is applied with the dog conscious in a normal standing position with the neck extended. The dog may require hand feeding initially but should later manage to take food from a shallow, raised bowl. Fluids need to be given by hand while the cast is worn. Animals in this series made good recoveries with conservative treatment even though follow up radiographs of some dogs showed quite marked displacement at the fracture site. The cervical neural canal is large relative to its contents and consequently affords greater leeway for compression than other areas of the spine.

In conclusion, fractures of the cervical vertebrae are uncommon; the prognosis for recovery is good with conservative treatment even when there is an alarming degree of displacement of the fragments. Surgical treatment carries distinct risks but can be justified in dogs where atlantoaxial subluxation results from fractures of the dens.

Fractures of the thoracic or lumbar vertebrae

Dogs presented with fractures of the thoracic or lumbar vertebrae immediately after road traffic accidents are usually paraplegic and have rigid extension of the forelimbs (Schiff Sherrington reflex). There is severe pain which can be localized to the area of the fracture and there may be obvious deformity in this region.

After a complete general and neurological examination radiographs should be taken of the spine in two planes. The types of fractures seen are:
1   Transverse fractures of the body of the vertebra.
2   Compression fractures in which the body of the vertebra is foreshortened and bony debris is displaced dorsally into the neural canal.
3   Fractures of the spinous and lateral processes: these do not involve the spinal cord directly and consequently there is no neurological deficit.

Subluxation and luxation of the vertebrae are also seen with or without concurrent fractures.

Prognosis for recovery following fractures or luxations of the thoracic or lumbar vertebrae is generally poor. If there is obvious displacement of the fragments or vertebrae then there is invariably cord transection or irreversible damage and the dog should be destroyed. Even when there is apparently little displacement of the vertebrae as in a sub-luxation, severe cord compression has often resulted because such injuries tend to occur in a 'whip lash' fashion, the vertebra being suddenly displaced dorsally in the accident and then sliding back into near normal alignment.

Surgical treatment should be reserved for the dog in which there is little displacement of the fragments or vertebrae. However, this is not quite so critical in the late lumbar region where there is relatively more room for the cord—cauda equina within the neural canal.

Treatment if it is to be of any value should be carried out

111

within hours of the accident. A laminectomy is performed over the site of cord compression to relieve pressure and allow inspection of the cord (Figs 134–137). (If there is evidence of gross tearing or contusion then the dog should be destroyed.) The vertebrae can be stabilized in a number of ways and these are illustrated in Figs 138–144.

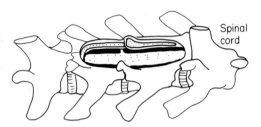

Fig. 134. Dorsal laminectomy of lumbar vertebrae: lateral view.

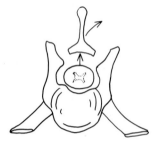

Fig. 135. Dorsal laminectomy of lumbar vertebrae: anterior view.

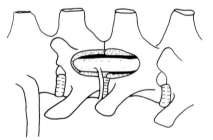

Fig. 136. Hemilaminectomy of lumbar vertebrae: lateral Spinal cord.

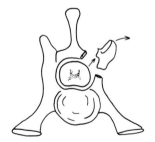

Fig. 137. Hemilaminectomy of lumbar vertebrae: anterior view.

Fig. 134 reproduced by permission of Trotter E.J. (1975). *Current Techniques in Small Animal Surgery*. Lea & Febiger. Philadelphia.

SURGICAL APPROACH

A dorsal midline skin incision is made over the fracture and the lumbodorsal fascia is incised. A periosteal elevator is used to separate the lumbar musculature from the spinous processes and the muscle attachments are severed from the

112

articular and accessory processes of the involved vertebrae. Blunt dissection and lateral retraction of muscle is continued down to the transverse processes or the rib heads of the vertebrae.

An alternative is the lateral approach as described for thoracolumbar disc fenestration (p. 103) and this is indicated if plate fixation (Fig. 143a) or transfixion pinning (Fig. 143b) of the vertebral bodies is to be performed.

After laminectomy and spinal fixation the dog will require careful nursing. Care of the paraplegic dog has already been described on page 102.

Methods of internal fixation for fractures of thoracic and lumbar vertebrae

Figures 138 and 139 show fixation using spinal plates applied to the dorsal spines of the vertebrae. Bolts are placed through the spine (Fig. 138, lateral view; Fig. 139, dorsal view) (Hoerlein 1971). Alternatively, plastic spinal plates can be used. Bolts are placed between the spinous processes and the plates grip the processes by friction (Fig. 140, dorsal view).

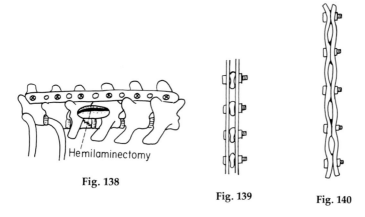

Hemilaminectomy

Fig. 138

Fig. 139   Fig. 140

Fixation using a U-shaped pin and wire sutures is illustrated in Figs 141 and 142 (Gage 1971). Plate fixation of the vertebral bodies (Swaim 1971, 1972) is shown in Fig. 143, and transfixion pinning of the vertebral bodies in Fig. 143b. (Gage 1969).

113

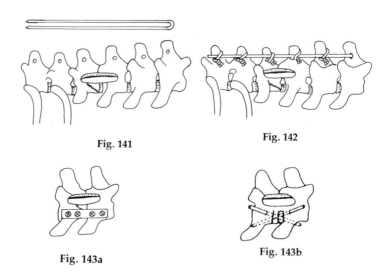

Fig. 141

Fig. 142

Fig. 143a

Fig. 143b

Figs 136 and 141–144 reproduced by permission of Swaim S.F. (1975). *Current Techniques in Small Animal Surgery*. Lea & Febiger. Philadelphia.

Cauda equia lesions (Denny *et al* 1982)

The cauda equina is described as the terminal portion of the spinal cord and adjacent nerve roots contained by the last three lumbar vertebrae, the sacrum and coccygeal vertebrae. It comprises nine nerve segments—one lumbar, three sacral and five coccygeal. The peripheral nerves of clinical importance which are derived from these segments include the sciatic, pudendal, pelvic and caudal nerves. The cauda equina syndrome (CES) has been defined as a neurological condition caused by compression, displacement or destruction of the cauda equina.

Lawson (1971) in an assessment of canine paraplegia, described the characteristic features of lesions at various levels of the spinal column. A lesion at the 6th lumbar vertebra produces complete sciatic nerve paralysis with total dysfunction of the hind legs except for the muscles supplied by the femoral and obturator nerves. A 7th lumbar vertebral lesion produces partial sciatic nerve paralysis and paralysis of the tail and bladder with sensory loss in the tail and around the anus. A third sacral vertebral lesion has the same effect as a 7th lumbar lesion except that the sciatic nerve is unaffected. Coccygeal vertebral lesions cause paralysis and loss of sensation of the tail only.

CAUSES OF CAUDA EQUINA SYNDROME
1 Lumbosacral spondylosis±disc protrusion | *In order of*
2 Lumbosacral discospondylitis. (Possible | *decreasing*
association with urinary tract infection, S. | *frequency*
aureus isolated from the disc most frequently.)
3 Fractures and dislocations.
4 Tumour.

CLINICAL FEATURES
1 Traumatic lesions—intense local pain paresis or paraplegia. Urinary retention
2 Discospondylitis—history of chronic urinary tract infection in some dogs. Stiffness or pain on rising. Hind leg lameness or weakness sometimes shifting from one leg to another. Urinary incontinence. A lateral radiograph of the lumbosacral junction shows destruction of end plates of vertebral bodies+much new bone formation. (Fig. 144a.)

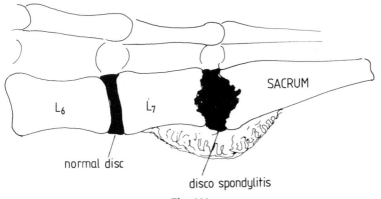

normal disc

disco spondylitis

Fig. 144a

3 Lumbosacral spondylosis±disc protrusion.
The larger breeds of dog are affected and the animals are presented with the same type of history as in the lumbosacral discospondylitis group. The most frequent clinical finding is lumbosacral pain, elicited by downward pres-

115

sure. Although hind leg lameness is most often unilateral, bilateral and sometimes shifting, hind leg lameness is seen. A few dogs show evidence of pain on palpation of the hips or stifle joints, but no other abnormalities except for muscle wasting are detected on clinical or radiological examination of the affected limb. Unilateral or bilateral hind leg paresis with a tendency to knuckle at the digits is occasionally seen. It is important to remember that lumbosacral spondylosis is a common incidental radiographic finding (Fig. 144b) in older dogs and is not necessarily of any clinical significance unless sufficient new bone is produced to impinge on the lumbar nerve roots.

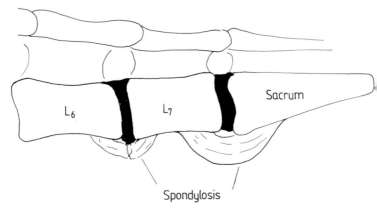

Fig. 144b

Treatment and Prognosis

Traumatic lesions of the last three lumbar vertebrae and the sacrum do not necessarily cause severe neurological deficits as the spinal canal in this region is large relative to its neural contents. Even with marked displacement good recoveries may follow reduction and internal fixation.

Dogs with discospondylitis generally respond well to prolonged antibiotic therapy (Ampicillin or Lincomycin). However, the response to conservative treatment in dogs with lumbosacral spondylosis or disc protrusion tends to be transient or incomplete. Surgical treatment by laminectomy (Fig. 144c) and facetectomy probably give better results in the long term.

116

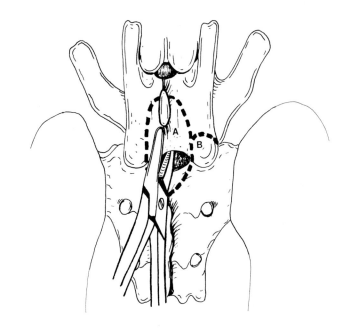

Dorsal view of lumlo-sacral junction
A – LAMINECTOMY
B – FACETECTOMY

Fig. 144c

REFERENCES

BENNETT D. & VAUGHAN L.C. (1976) The use of muscle relocation techniques in the treatment of peripheral nerve injuries in dogs and cats. *J. small Anim. Pract.* **17**, 99.

BOJRAB M.J. (1971) Disc disease. *Vet. Rec.* **89**, 37.

CAMERON STEWART W., BAKER G.J. & LEE R. (1975) Temporomandibular subluxation in the dog: a case report. *J. small Anim. Pract.* **16**, 345.

DE LAHUNTA A. & ALEXANDER J.W. (1976) Ischaemic myelopathy secondary to presumed fibrocartila ginous emboli in 9 dogs. *J. Am. Anim. Hosp. Ass.* **12**, 37.

DE LAHUNTA A. (1977) *Veterinary Neuroanatomy and Clinical Neurology.* Philadelphia, Saunders, pp. 191–338.

DENNY H.R. (1978) The surgical treatment of cervical disc protrusions in the dog: a review of 40 cases. *J. small Anim. Pract.* **19**, 251.

DENNY H.R. (1978) The lateral fenestration of canine thoracolumbar disc protrusions: a review of 30 cases. *J. small Anim. Pract.* **19**, 259.

DENNY H.R., GIBBS Christine & GASKELL C.J. (1977) Cervical spondylopathy in the dog: a review of 35 cases. *J. small Anim. Pract.* **18**, 117.

DENNY H.R. (1982) The lateral fenestration of thorocolumbar disc protusion in the dog. *The Veterinary Annual*. p. 169 22nd Ed. Scientechnic, Bristol.

DENNY H.R., GIBBS C. & HOLT P.E. (1982) The diagnosis and treatment of cauda equina lesions in the dog. *J. small Anim. Pract.* **23**, 425.

DUNCAN I.D. & GRIFFITHS I.R. (1981) Canine giant axonal neuropathy; some aspects of its clinical, pathological and cooperative features. *J. small Anim. Pract.* **22**, 491.

FLO G.L. & BRINKER W.O. (1975) Lateral fenestration of thoracolumbar discs. *J. Am. Anim. Hosp. Ass.* **11**, 619.

FUNKQUIST B. (1962) Thoracolumbar disc protrusions with severe cord compression in the dog. *Acta Vet. Scan.* **3**, 000.

GAGE E.D. (1975) Atlanto-axial subluxation. In: *Current Techniques in Small Animal Surgery*, Bojrab M.J. (ed.). Lea & Febiger, Philadelphia.

GAGE E.D. (1969) A new method of spinal fixation in the dog. *Vet. Med. Small Anim. Clin.* **64**, 295.

GAGE E.D. (1971) Surgical repair of spinal fractures in small breed dogs. *Vet. Med. Small Anim. Clin.* **66**, 295.

GAGE E.D. & SMALLWOOD J.E. (1970) Surgical repair of atlantoaxial subluxation in a dog. *Vet. Med. Small Anim. Clin.* **65**, 692.

GAGE E.D. (1968) Surgical repair of a fractured cervical spine in the dog. *J. Am. Vet. Med. Assoc.* **153**, 1407.

GEARY J.C., OLIVER J.E. & HOERLEIN B.F. (1967) Atlanto-axial subluxation in the canine. *J. small Anim. Pract.* **8**, 577.

GRIFFITHS I.R., DUNCAN I.D. & BARKER J. (1980) A progressive axonopathy of Boxer dogs affecting the central and peripheral nervous system. *J. small Anim. Pract.* **21**, 29.

GRIFFITHS I.R. & DUNCAN I.D. (1979) Distal denervating disease; a degenerative neuropathy of the distal motor ancon in dogs. *J. small Anim. Pract.* **20**, 579.

GRIFFITHS I.R. & DUNCAN I.D. (1975) Chronic degenerative radiculomyelopathy in the dog. *J. small Anim. Pract.* **16**, 461.

GRIFFITHS I.R. (1972) Some aspects of the pathogenesis and diagnosis of lumbar disc protrusion in the dog. *J. small Anim. Pract.* **13**, 439.

GRIFFITHS I.R., DUNCAN I.D. & LAWSON D.D. (1974) Avulsion of the brachial plexus—2 clinical aspects. *J. small Anim. Pract.* **15**, 177.

HANSEN H.J. (1952) *Acta Orthop. Scan.* Suppl. **11**, 1–117.

HAYES M.A., CREIGHTON S.R., BOYSEN B.G. & HOLFIELD N. (1978) Acute necrotizing myelopathy from nucleus pulposus embolism of arteries and veins in large dogs with early disc degeneration. *J. Am. Anim. Hosp. Ass.* **173**, 289.

HOERLEIN B.F. (1956) Further evaluation of the treatment of disc protrusion paraplegia in the dog. *J. Am. Vet. Med. Ass.* **129**, 495.

HOERLEIN B.F. (1971) *Canine Neurology—Diagnosis and Treatment*, 2nd edn. W.B. Saunders Co, Philadelphia.

KNECHT C.D. & SCHILLER A.G. (1974) *Canine Surgery*, 2nd edn. American Vet. Publications, Wheaton, Illinois.

LADDS P., GUFFY M., BLAUCH B. & SPLITTER G. (1970) *Congenital odontoid separation in Two Dogs. J. small Anim. Pract.* **12**, 463.

LAWSON D.D. (1957) Fixation of mandibular fractures in the dog and cat by transfixing pinning. *Vet. Rec.* **69**, 1029.

LAWSON D.D. (1963) *Br. Vet. J.* **119**, 492.

LEONARD E.P. (1971) *Orthopaedic Surgery of the Dog and Cat,* 2nd edn. W.B. Saunders Co, Philadelphia.

OLIVER E. & LEWIS E. (1973) Lesions of the atlas and axis in dogs. *J. Am. Anim. Hosp. Assoc.* **9,** 304.

OLIVER J.E. (1975) Craniotomy, craniectomy and skull fractures; in *Current Techniques in Small Animal Surgery,* ed. Bojrab M.J. Lea & Febiger, Philadelphia, p. 359.

OLSSON S.E. & HANSEN H.J. (1952) Cervical disc protrusion in the dog. *J. Am. Vet. Med. Ass.* **121,** 361.

PALMER A.C. (1965) *Introduction to Animal Neurology,* 1st edn. Blackwell Scientific Publications, Oxford.

READ R.A., ROBINS G.M. & CARLISLE C.H. (1983) Caudal cervical spondylo-myelopathy (Wobbler syndrome) in the dog; a review of 30 cases. *J. small Anim. Pract.* **24,** 605.

ROBINS G.N. (1976) Dropped jaw—mandibular neurapraxia in the dog. *J. small Anim. Pract.* **17,** 753.

ROBINS G.N. & GRANDAGE J. (1977) Temporomandibular joint dysplasia and open mouth jaw locking in the dog. *J. Am. Med. Ass.* **171,** 1072.

ROUSE G.P. (1979) Cervical spine stabilization with methylmethacrylate. *Vet. Surg.* **8,** 1.

RUSSELL R.W. & GRIFFITHS R.C. (1968) Recurrence of cervical disc syndrome in surgically and conservatively treated dogs. *J. Am. Vet. Med. Ass.* **153,** 1412.

SEEMANN C.W. (1968) A lateral approach for thoracolumbar disc fenestra-tion. *Mod. Vet. Pract.* **49,** 73.

SEEMANN C.W. (1980) Anatomic orientation for lateral thoracolumbar disc fenestration. *Vet. Med. Small Anim. Clin.* **75,** 1865.

SPELLMAN G. (1972) *Vet. Med. SAC* **67,** 1213.

STONE E.A., BETTS C.W. & CHAMBERS J.N. (1979) Cervical fractures in the dog: a literature and case review. *J. Am. Anim. Hosp. Assoc.* **15,** 463.

SUMNER SMITH G. & DINGWALL J.S. (1971) The plating of mandibular frac-tures in the dog. *Vet. rec.* **88,** 595.

SUMNER SMITH G. & DINGWALL J.S. (1973) The plating of mandibular frac-tures in giant dogs. *Vet. Rec.* **92,** 39.

SUMNER SMITH G. (1974) Personal communication.

SWAIM S.F. (1971) Vertebral body plating for spinal immobilization. *J. Am. Vet. Med. Ass.* **158,** 1683.

SWAIM S.F. (1972) Surgical correction of a spinal fracture in a day. *J. Am. Vet Med. Ass.* **158,** 1683.

SWAIM F. (1975) Evaluation of four techniques of cervical spinal fixation in dogs. *J. Am. Vet. Med. Assoc.* **166,** 1080.

WEINMANN J.P. & SICHER H. (1955) *Bone and Bones: Fundamentals of Bone Biology,* 2nd edn. London, Kimpton, p. 309.

WHITBREAD T.J. (1981) *Personal communication.*

WINSTANLEY E.W. (1976) Fractures of the skull. *Vet. Annual,* **16,** 151. John Wright & Sons, Bristol.

WOLFF E.F. (1974) *Vet. Med. SAC* **69,** 859.

WORTHMAN R.P. (1957) Demonstration of specific nerve paralyses in the Dog. *J. Am. Vet. Med. Ass.* **131,** 174.

Chapter 4
The Forelimb

Examination of the dog with foreleg lameness

The following points should be noted in the history:
1 Breed of dog.
2 Age.
3 Speed of onset of lameness—gradual or sudden. If the onset was sudden, has the animal been involved in an accident, fall or other trauma?
4 Is lameness constant or intermittent? If intermittent, is lameness worse after exercise or rest?
5 Has the dog had any other problems?
6 In road traffic accident cases fractures or dislocations may be obvious but it is important not to overlook injuries to the chest or urinary tract.

The history will often give good hints towards diagnosis. The developmental disorders tend to be seen in certain breeds of dog and generally cause a gradual onset of lameness in animals under a year of age. A sudden onset of lameness indicates a traumatic episode; common causes include a sprained joint, foreign body in the foot and bite wounds.

Dogs with fractures or dislocations will usually carry the affected leg. The clinical features of a fracture include:
1 Abnormal mobility of bone where no joint exists.
2 Deformity, i.e. local swelling, angulation and shortening of the limb.
3 Crepitus—a grating noise as the bone ends rub together.
4 Pain.

In a dislocation, unlike a fracture where the limb 'waves in the breeze' from the fracture site, characteristic postures are adopted as a result of joint displacement. Joint mobility is restricted and painful but crepitus is not generally as obvious as in a fracture.

Dislocations and ligamentous ruptures tend to be seen in mature dogs over 1 year of age. The same trauma in immature animals is more likely to cause a fracture or separation of an epiphysis.

The common, or well–recognised causes of foreleg lameness, are listed below and should be kept in mind when the clinical examination is carried out.

DEVELOPMENTAL DISORDERS CAUSING FORELEG LAMENESS

Shoulder:	Osteochondritis dissecans	Giant breeds, especially Irish Wolfhounds, Pyrenean Mountain Dogs, Great Danes, but can affect any large dog from Labrador–size upwards.
Elbow:	Ununited anconeal process	Alsatian, Basset Hound.
	Osteochondritis dissecans	Labrador, Retriever, Rottweiler.
	Ununited coronoid process	
Carpus:	Lateral deviation due to growth disturbances of the radius and ulna.	Great Dane, Irish Wolfhound.

TRAUMATIC CONDITIONS OF THE FORELIMB

Shoulder:	Dislocations	Gross instability— lateral dislocation of humeral head most often.
Humeral shaft Fractures:		Distal third mainly, spiral or oblique, often comminuted.
Elbow:	Dislocation	Radial head dislocates laterally, forearm swung out laterally, held forward and

122

		supinated.
Condylar fractures		Spaniels are particularly prone to this injury. Lateral condyle fractures most frequently, also 'Y' and 'T' fractures.
	Fracture of the olecranon	
Fractures of shaft of radius and ulna:		Generally transverse and involve distal third.
Carpus:	Fracture of accessory carpal bone.	Racing Greyhound.
	Hyperextension of carpus due to rupture of plantar ligaments.	
Metacarpus:		Fractures and crush injuries common.
Greyhound toe injuries:	Interphalangeal subluxations and dislocations.	Left foot most frequently involved.
	Fractures— phalanges and sesamoids.	
	'Knocked up toe'	

CONDITIONS CAUSING A GRADUAL ONSET OF
LAMENESS: OLDER DOGS

Brachial plexus tumour.
Bicipital tenosynovitis: shoulder.
Osteosarcoma: proximal humerus.
Osteoarthritis: elbow.
Osteosarcoma: distal radius.
Osteoarthritis: carpus.

Physical examination

Look at the dog standing, assess weight bearing and look for evidence of muscle wasting. The spine of the scapula becomes more prominent in chronic foreleg lameness and the greater trochanter of the femur becomes more prominent in chronic hind leg lameness. Note any joint deformity. Observe the animal's gait when walking, trotting and running, both in a straight line and in a circle. Assess the degree of lameness and differentiate lameness from ataxia or paresis.

Most larger dogs feel more secure and behave better if examined on the floor. Small dogs are obviously easier to handle and examine on a table. The owner or assistant should hold the dog's head firmly from the contralateral side to the leg being examined. Run your hands down both front legs, compare the affected leg with the normal one, check for muscle wasting, joint swelling and deformity. Check the nails and pads; in chronic lameness the nails will be long and there will be little wear of the pads compared with the normal foot. Alternatively, the dog with foreleg paresis will often have excessive wear of the nails through dragging the toes or knuckling at the digits. Each joint should be checked systematically. The shoulder is fully extended. The leg should be gripped *above* the elbow with one hand and pulled forward, while the other hand is placed over the anterior aspect of the shoulder and used to push the joint caudally. Remember that extension of the shoulder naturally tends to extend the elbow and it is possible to confuse pain arising from either joint. A sudden onset of shoulder pain is most frequently caused by strain of the shoulder muscles and lameness will resolve provided adequate rest is given. If an immature dog of the larger breeds has pain on extension of the shoulder and the onset of lameness is gradual, then the most likely cause is osteochondritis dissecans. A limited range of shoulder flexion sometimes associated with pain is seen in dogs with bicipital tenosynovitis or contracture of the extensor muscles of the shoulder. A limited range of shoulder movement is also seen in small breeds of dog with congenital dislocation. The proximal humerus is a common site for osteosarcoma formation and the lesion causes a hard, painful swelling. It is also worth checking the axilla for tumour formation in older animals.

The elbow is checked next. One hand is cupped behind

124

the olecranon and the other is used to grip the forearm and gradually extend the elbow. Pain on extension is a feature of ununited anconeal process, osteochondritis dissecans and ununited coronoid process. If either of the last two conditions are present pain can be increased by supinating the forearm while extending the elbow. Ununited anconeal process causes an increase in synovial fluid production and a fluctuating swelling develops caudal to the humeral condyles. All three conditions if untreated cause osteoarthritis, the elbow joint becomes thickened with a limited range of flexion, crepitus and there is a varying degree of pain on manipulation.

Condylar fractures of the humerus cause obvious pain and crepitus in the elbow. Fracture of the lateral condyle occurs most frequently. Lateral support for the joint is lost and the distal humerus can be palpated subluxating medially in relation to the radius and ulna. By comparison palpation of the elbow in a dog with an intercondylar fracture ('Y' or 'T' fracture) reveals total disruption in the continuity of the distal humerus. Dislocation of the elbow results in a limited range of painful joint movement and the forearm is held forward abducted and supinated.

The main movements of the carpus are flexion and extension. Hyperextension is seen in Alsatian puppies occasionally and is associated with laxity of the carpal flexor tendons and ligaments. Traumatic hyperextension is seen in mature dogs with rupture of the plantar ligaments of the carpus. In the racing Greyhound feel the accessory carpal bone; chip fractures are common and give rise to pain on flexion and extension of the joint. Normally there is little medial or lateral movement of the carpus unless there has been damage to the collateral ligaments. Lateral deviation of the carpus and foot (carpal valgus) is seen in immature giant breeds of dog due to growth disturbances of the radius and ulna. Thickening and pain in the carpus is usually due to osteoarthritis. However, the distal radius is a common site for osteosarcoma formation. Feel the metacarpal bones and, in the racing Greyhound, particular care should be taken over the palpation of the toes as injuries are common. Finally, look at the nails for damage and check the pads for cuts, bruising or foreign bodies.

If the physical examination of the lame dog causes obvious pain further manipulation if necessary, should be done under general anaesthesia. The radiographic examination is undertaken next. The most useful views are:

Shoulder: lateral radiograph

Elbow: flexed lateral and A.P. radiographs

Carpus: A.P. and lateral radiographs.

If joint is unstable the lateral radiograph is taken first with the carpus flexed and secondly with the joint extended.

Other procedures such as (a) the aspiration and examination of synovial fluid, (b) special serological tests for conditions like rheumatoid arthritis, systemic lupus erythematosus or toxoplasmosis, and (c) exploratory arthrotomy may be necessary to determine the cause of lameness.

If the initial findings are negative the dog is rested and treated symptomatically. Radiographic examination is repeated 4–6 weeks later if lameness has not resolved. The repeat radiograph is particularly useful when initial findings were suggestive but not conclusive for osteosarcoma formation.

The shoulder

The shoulder is an enarthrodial joint (Figs. 145 and 146).

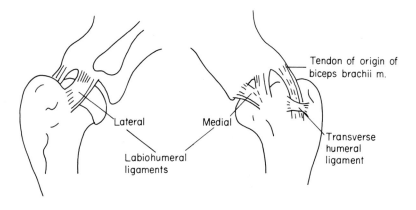

Fig. 145. Shoulder, lateral view.　　Fig. 146. Shoulder, medial view.

Although there are weak medial and lateral labio humeral ligaments present, the joint is mainly supported by the surrounding muscles. Support is provided cranially by the supraspinatus muscle laterally by the infraspinatus muscle, ventrolaterally by the teres minor muscle and medially by the subscapularis muscle (Fig. 147). The tendon of the biceps brachii muscle crosses the anteromedial aspect of the joint and is retained in the bicipital groove of the humerus by the transverse humeral ligament (Fig. 146).

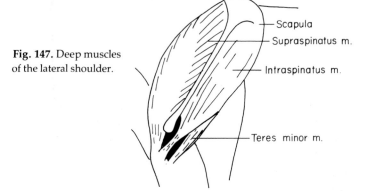

Fig. 147. Deep muscles of the lateral shoulder.

- Scapula
- Supraspinatus m.
- Intraspinatus m.
- Teres minor m.

Figs. 145–147 reproduced by permission of Miller M.E. (1952) A Guide to the Dissection of the Dog. Edwards Brothers Inc. Michigan.

The superficial muscles of the shoulder are illustrated in Fig. 148.

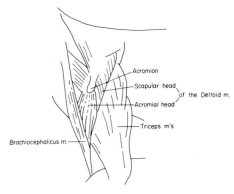

- Acromion
- Scapular head
- of the Deltoid m.
- Acromial head
- Triceps m's
Brachiocephalicus m.

Fig. 148

127

There are few 'danger points' in the exposure of the shoulder but structures to recognize and avoid include:

1   A branch of the cephalic vein which runs just cranial to the joint.

2   The circumflex humeral artery and vein and the axillary nerve caudal to the joint.

3   The suprascapular nerve which runs around the neck of the scapula.

Conditions which can affect the canine shoulder joint are summarized in Fig. 149.

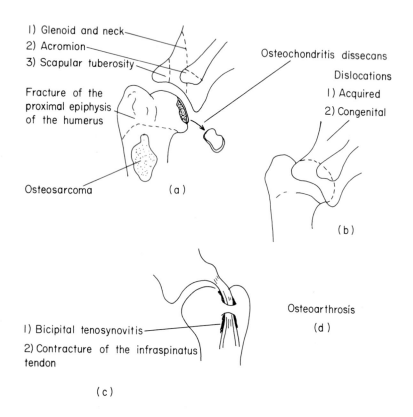

Fig. 149. (a) Fractures of the scapula (1, 2 and 3); (b) shoulder dysplasia, acquired and congenital dislocation. (c) muscle injuries include bicipital tenosynovitis and contracture of the infraspinatus tendon; and (d) osteoarthritis.

Traumatic conditions of the shoulder

Fractures of the scapula (Cheli 1976; Caywood *et al* 1977; Holt 1978; Piermattei & Greeley 1979)

The scapula with its blade–like structure, lateral supporting muscle mass and proximity to the chest wall is well protected against trauma. Consequently, scapular fractures are uncommon. Generally, the fragments are well supported by the adjacent tissues and this, together with the cancellous nature of the bone ensures that the majority of scapular fractures will heal well with conservative treatment. An elastoplast support bandage is applied around the shoulder and chest for four weeks. The exceptions which should be treated surgically include intra–articular fractures, avulsion fractures and grossly displaced fractures of the blade and neck.

DISPLACED FRACTURES OF THE SCAPULAR BLADE AND SPINE

The supraspinatus and infraspinatus muscles are reflected to reveal the fracture site. Wire sutures are a popular method of fixation. However, a plate will provide better stability. If the screws are to achieve maximum purchase in the bone, the plate should be placed in the angle formed between the spine and body (Fig. 151). An ASIF semi-tubular plate fits the angle well if it is applied upside down with the convex side of the plate towards the bone.

FRACTURE OF THE ACROMION

The acromion is distracted by the deltoid muscle following fracture. Fixation is simply achieved using one of two wire sutures (Fig. 152).

FRACTURES OF THE SCAPULAR NECK AND GLENOID

(Figs. 153a,b,c)

Osteotomy of the acromion is carried out to allow ventral reflection of the acromial head of the deltoid. (The osteotomy is repaired during wound closure with wire sutures as shown in Fig. 152). The underlying supraspinatus muscle is retracted cranially. The tendon of insertion of the infra-

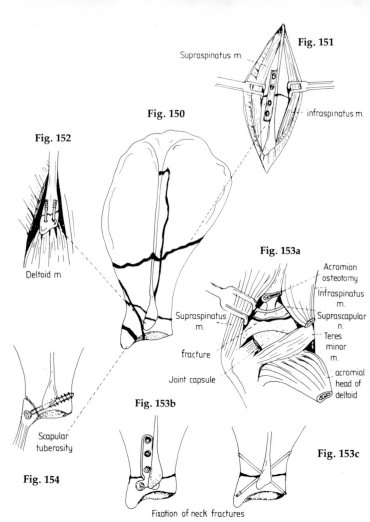

Fig. 151

Supraspinatus m.

infraspinatus m.

Fig. 150

Fig. 152

Deltoid m.

Fig. 153a

Acromion osteotomy

Infraspinatus m.

Suprascapular n.

Teres minor m.

acromial head of deltoid

Supraspinatus m.

fracture

Joint capsule

Fig. 153b

Scapular tuberosity

Fig. 154

Fig. 153c

Fixation of neck fractures

spinatus muscle is cut and the muscle is reflected caudally to complete exposure of the scapular neck, suprascapular nerve and joint capsule. The nerve must be carefully protected during fracture reduction and fixation. Transverse fractures of the scapular neck are stabilized using a small ASIF mini 'T' plate (Fig. 153b) or two Kirschner wires (Fig. 153c). Lag screw fixation is used for sagittal fractures of the scapular neck which extend into the glenoid. The joint capsule should be opened during exposure of the fracture to check that accurate anatomical reduction of the fragments is achieved.

AVULSION OF THE SCAPULAR TUBEROSITY

The scapular tuberosity develops as a separate ossification

centre which fuses with the scapula when the dog reaches approximately 5 months of age. Avulsion of the tuberosity occasionally occurs in immature dogs, the fracture extends through the growth plate and the fragment is distracted by the pull of the biceps tendon (Fig. 154). The fracture is exposed by retracting the brachiocephalicus muscle cranially to reveal the greater tuberosity of the humerus and the insertion of the supraspinatus muscle. The shoulder is rotated laterally and the scapular tuberosity exposed by blunt dissection medial to the insertion of the supraspinatus muscle. The fracture is stabilized with a lag screw (preferably cancellous) or a tension band wire (Fig. 154).

In a chronic avulsion fracture, reduction may be impossible due to contracture of the biceps brachii muscle. Under these circumstances, the scapular tuberosity is excised and the biceps tendon sutured to the transverse humeral ligament.

FRACTURES INVOLVING THE PROXIMAL HUMERAL EPIPHYSIS AND METAPHYSIS

Fractures of the proximal humerus can be divided into intra–articular fractures in which there is involvement of the humeral head and/or tubercles, and extra–articular fractures where fracture occurs either through the proximal growth plate of the humerus with separation of the epiphysis (epiphysiolysis) or through the metaphyseal region.

Intra–articular fractures are rare, they occur in immature animals and the fracture extends through the growth plate. Exposure of the humeral head is described elsewhere. Fixation of the fracture is achieved with two Kirschner wires driven through the lateral aspect of the greater tuberosity and on into the humeral head (Fig. 155a). Conversely the wires can be introduced through the articular surface of the humerus but the ends must be countersunk with a nail punch to allow normal shoulder movement.

FRACTURE–SEPARATION OF THE PROXIMAL EPIPHYSIS OF THE HUMERUS

This is a rare injury which occurs in immature dogs. Considerable trauma is needed to separate the epiphysis and

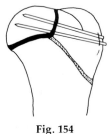

Fig. 154

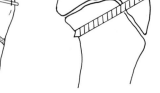

Fig. 155

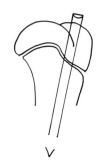

V

Fig. 156

there is usually gross anterior displacement of the epiphysis in relation to the metaphysis. Open reduction is necessary in most cases. A longitudinal skin incision is made over the antero–lateral aspect of the proximal humerus. The brachiocephalicus muscle is retracted cranially to expose the fracture. The epiphysis is grasped with small AO reduction forceps (Straumann, G.B. Ltd) and with the aid of a periosteal elevator the epiphysis is levered back into its normal position. Generally, stability is good once reduction is achieved and this can be maintained with a lag screw in dogs approaching maturity (Fig. 155) or an intramedullary pin in puppies (Fig. 156). Healing should occur within 4–6 weeks. Premature closure of the growth plate may occur as a result of the initial trauma but this is of doubtful significance unless it happens in a pup under 6 months of age. The lag screw or intramedullary pin is removed as soon as fracture healing is complete.

Dislocation of the shoulder

CONGENITAL DISLOCATION (Vaughan & Clayton Jones 1969)

The condition is rare and is usually seen in toy breeds of dogs. The humeral head luxates medially in most cases and the glenoid cavity is deformed and convex. Both shoulder joints may be affected. There is no treatment but as these animals are usually small and light they are not greatly incapacitated by the deformity.

132

(Vaughan 1967; Ball 1968; Campbell 1968; Leighton 1969; De Angelis & Schwartz 1970; Hohn 1971)

Acquired dislocation of the shoulder is uncommon. The humeral head may luxate medially or laterally. Lateral dislocation is seen most often. Manipulation of the shoulder reveals gross instability and spontaneous reduction often occurs when the dog is positioned for radiographic examination.

Stabilization of the joint to prevent recurrence of the dislocation can be a real problem. In fresh dislocations closed reduction and shoulder support with body cast (Fig. 34a) for 3 weeks may prevent redislocation, however in the majority of dogs some form of internal fixation is necessary. Techniques include:

1   Suturing the torn joint capsule and damaged shoulder muscles.

2   Braided nylon, terylene or a strip of skin can be threaded through a tunnel in the spine of the scapula and then down through the greater tuberosity on the lateral side of the joint in a figure of eight pattern (Fig. 157) to form a prosthetic ligament.

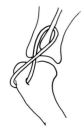

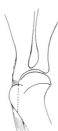

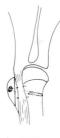

Fig. 157   Fig. 158a   Fig. 158b

3   The biceps tendon can be transposed medially or laterally (depending on the direction of the dislocation) to serve as a collateral ligament (Figs. 158a,b). Osteotomy of the greater tuberosity is necessary to permit lateral transposition of the tendon.

4   A simple and effective method of re–stabilizing the shoulder following dislocation in any direction is shown in Figs. 159 a–e. In a medium sized dog, a double strand of No.

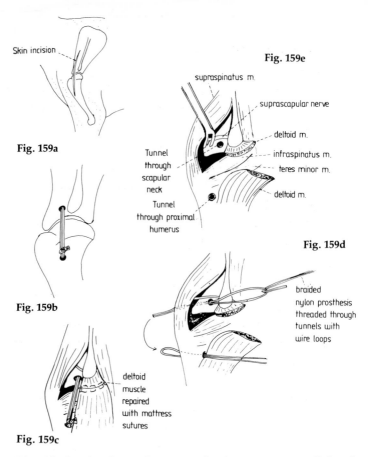

Skin incision

Fig. 159a

Fig. 159b

deltoid
muscle
repaired
with mattress
sutures

Fig. 159c

Fig. 159e

supraspinatus m.

suprascapular nerve

deltoid m.

infraspinatus m.

teres minor m.

deltoid m.

Tunnel
through
scapular
neck

Tunnel
through proximal
humerus

Fig. 159d

braided
nylon prosthesis
threaded through
tunnels with
wire loops

7 braided nylon is used as a prosthesis to create a medial and lateral collateral ligament for the shoulder (Fig. 159b). A skin incision is made directly over the joint (Fig. 159a). The acromial head of the deltoid is sectioned about 1 cm from its origin and the muscle belly is reflected to reveal the infraspinatus and supraspinatus muscles (Fig. 159c). The supraspinatus muscle and the suprascapular nerve are retracted to expose the neck of the scapula. A tunnel is drilled through the scapular neck and a second tunnel is drilled through the proximal humerus. The shoulder is rotated laterally and wire loops are used to thread the braided nylon from lateral to medial through the scapular tunnel and then from medial to lateral through the humeral tunnel. The joint capsule is repaired and then the ends of the nylon prosthesis are tied. A support bandage is applied round the shoulder for 2 weeks following surgery.

Shoulder dysplasia (Evans 1968)

Shoulder dysplasia resulting in excessive joint laxity is occasionally encountered in the dog. The condition has been described n 3½ year old Collie (Hanlon 1964) and a 10 month old Labrador (Evans 1968).

Muscle and tendon injuries

Two specific muscle and tendon injuries of the shoulder are recognized. These are bicipital tenosynovitis and contracture of the infraspinatus muscle or supraspinatus muscle.

Bicipital tenosynovitis

This condition is usually seen in older dogs of the larger breeds which are presented with chronic foreleg lameness. The range of shoulder movement may be limited and there is pain on flexion of the joint. Damage to the biceps tendon results in an inflammatory reaction and the end result is fibrous adhesions between tendon and its sheath. Evidence of new bone formation within the bicipital groove may be seen on a lateral radiograph of the shoulder.

Intra—articular injection of methylprednisolone(depomedrone Upjohn) should alleviate lameness, but strict rest should be given for 4 weeks also. Recurrences of lameness are to be suspected.

Contracture of the infraspinatus or supraspinatus muscle
(Hufford *et al.* 1975; Vaughan 1979)

Contracture of the infraspinatus muscle is an occasional cause of foreleg lameness in the dog. Contracture of the supraspinatus muscle occurs even less frequently and gives similar signs. Working dogs are usually affected and have an acute onset of lameness at exercise. Although use of the affected limb is regained within two or three weeks, an abnormal action persists characterised by lateral circumduction of the distal limb with a rapid flip—like extension of the paw when the foot is advanced. Range of shoulder flexion is limited and there is atrophy of the supra— and infraspinatus muscles. On full flexion of the leg the forearm swings out laterally from the body instead of moving forward in a straight line. A. P. radiographs of the shoulder may show that the gap between the acromion and the greater tuberosity is reduced on the side of contracture (Fig. 160b). Normal limb function is rapidly restored by tenotomy of the contracted infraspinatus or supraspinatus tendon of insertion.

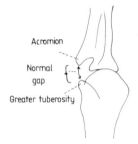

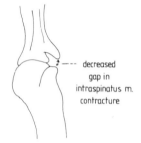

AP Normal shoulder   **Fig. 160a**   **Fig. 160b**

Osteochondritis dissecans (Craig 1965; Birkeland 1967; Griffiths 1968; Clayton Jones & Vaughan 1968, 1970; Smith & Stowater 1975; Olsson 1975, 1976)

Osteochondritis dissecans (OCD) is a disease of articular cartilage characterized by focal separation of articular cartilage and subchondral bone. The disease can affect the shoulder, elbow, stifle or hock but it is most frequently diagnosed as a cause of shoulder lameness. The condition is often bilateral but generally only one pair of joints is involved. Olsson (1976) has shown tht OCD is due to abnormal enchondral ossification. Typically, the lesion is found in the caudal part of the humeral head (Fig. 161a). Here the articular cartilage becomes thicker than normal because enchondral ossification does not keep pace with normal cartilaginous growth. The deeper layers of chondrocytes die and a zone of chondromalacia is formed. Modelling of the joint surface may be delayed giving flattening (Fig. 161b) or more typically cleavage occurs through the zone of chondromalacia and the overlying flap of cartilage becomes detached (Fig. 161c). The flap eventually comes to lie in the caudal part of the joint below the

136

humeral head. In this position the flap does not interfere with joint function. The flap may survive on synovial fluid, grow and ossify and it is then referred to as a joint mouse (Fig. 161c). The erosion in the humeral head heals by fibrocartilage formation.

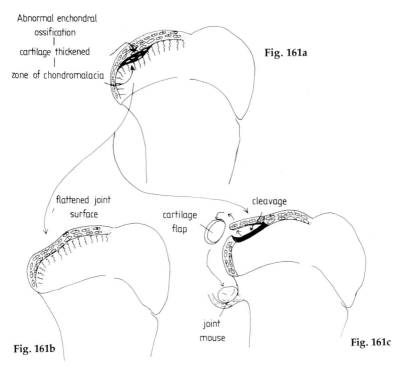

Abnormal enchondral ossification
cartilage thickened
zone of chondromalacia

Fig. 161a

flattened joint surface

cartilage flap

cleavage

joint mouse

Fig. 161b

Fig. 161c

A number of factors play a part in the development of osteochondritis dissecans lesions. These include genetic factors, feeding, exercise and trauma. Trauma is thought to be important in the aetiology of osteochondritis dissecans because lesions are invariably found in those areas of articular cartilage which are particularly prone to concussion. It has been shown that the caudal part of the humeral head where the lesion is found, is prone to concussion both when the shoulder is in the flexed and extended positions.

The large and giant breeds of dog, especially the Pyrenean Mountain Dog, Irish Wolfhound and Great Dane are affected most frequently by osteochondritis dissecans of the shoulder. Male dogs, presumably because of their greater weight, are affected more often than females. The condition is bilateral in just over 50% of cases. OCD is a disease of the *immature* dog (no matter which joint is involved) and causes a gradual onset of lameness before the dog reaches a year of age. The average age at the onset of lameness is 5 months. Lameness tends to be intermittent in nature and is often worse after exercise or immediately the dog gets up from rest. The main finding on clinical examination is pain on extension of the shoulder. Later the shoulder muscles become wasted and the spine of the scapula becomes more prominent.

A lateral radiograph of the joint will usually confirm the diagnosis. In doubtful cases two further lateral radiographs are taken, one with the head of the humerus rotated medially and the other with the humeral head rotated laterally. Osteochondritis dissecans affects the caudal humeral head and in positive cases flattening or an erosion will be seen in the subchondral bone of this region (Fig.

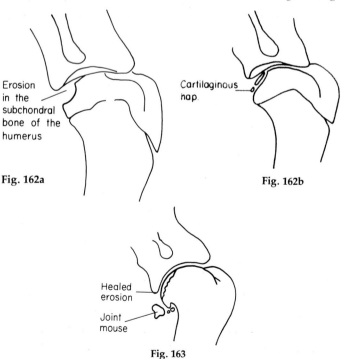

Erosion in the subchondral bone of the humerus

Fig. 162a

Cartilaginous flap.

Fig. 162b

Healed erosion

Joint mouse

Fig. 163

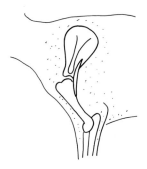

Fig. 164

162a). The overlying flap of articular cartilage is radiolucent but with time it becomes calcified and appears as a fine white line over the erosion (Fig. 162b). In chronic cases a joint mouse may be seen. There may be irregularity of the humeral head at the site of the original erosion and osteophyte develop especially around the caudal margins of the joint (Fig. 163). Although dogs are usually clinically lame on one leg only, the condition affects both shoulders in approximately 50% of cases; consequently both joints are radiographed as a routine.

Treatment
The majority of dogs with OCD of the shoulder would eventually recover with conservative treatment. However, the recovery period is prolonged (several months) and healing may be complicated by osteoarthrosis in the joint. Conservative treatment (restricted exercise and analgesics) is used in the early stages of the disease, especially if the lesion is small on radiographic examination. If lameness shows no signs of resolution within 6 weeks and there is definite radiographic evidence of OCD, then surgical treatment should be recommended. An arthrotomy is performed, the cartilaginous flap removed and the erosion in the humeral head curetted. An interesting feature of OCD is that shoulder pain persists until the cartilaginous flap becomes detached. Once this happens, pain rapidly disappears and lameness resolves. Some veterinarians favour an aggressive form of conservative treatment in which the

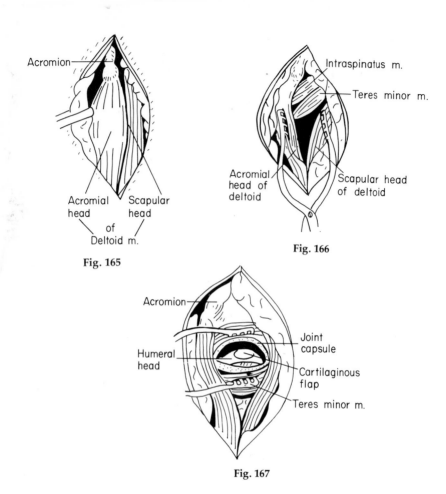

Fig. 165

Fig. 166

Fig. 167

dog is encouraged to exercise, run up and down slopes and
the shoulder is forcibly manipulated. The rationale of these
manoeuvres is to cause early detachment of the
cartilaginous flap.

SURGICAL TECHNIQUE

A curved skin incision is made over the shoulder just caudal
to the scapular spine. The subcutaneous fat and fascia are
retracted to expose the acromion and the acromial head and
scapular head of the deltoid muscle (Fig. 165). The two
heads of the deltoid are separated and retracted to expose
the infraspinatus and the teres minor muscles (Fig. 166).

The infraspinatus and the teres minor muscles are

140

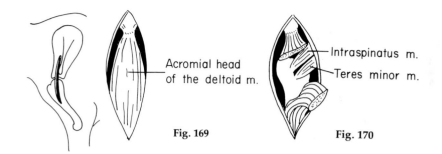

Acromial head
of the deltoid m.

Fig. 169

Intraspinatus m.

Teres minor m.

Fig. 170

Fig. 168

separated and retracted to expose the joint capsule (Figs. 166 and 167). A transverse incision is made in the joint capsule to reveal the articular surface of the humeral head and the osteochondritis dissecans lesion. The flap of cartilage is removed and the underlying erosion in the subchondral bone curetted. The joint is flushed out with saline solution to remove any remaining fragments. Closure of the wound is routine.

An alternative approach to the shoulder is illustrated in Figs. 168–170. This approach is more traumatic but provides better exposure and is ideal for the surgeon who only occasionally operates on the shoulder.

A skin incision is made over the spine of the scapula and extended down over the proximal third of the humerus. The acromial head of the deltoid is exposed and the origin of the muscle is transected approximately 2 cm from the acromion. The muscle is reflected to reveal the infraspinatus and teres minor muscles which are separated to expose the joint capsule. The arthrotomy is then performed as described above.

After surgery, exercise is restricted to walking on a leash for one month. Most dogs are less lame than before the operation within the month and should be sound within three months. In dogs with bilateral lesions a 6 week interval is left between each arthrotomy. The second operation is seldom necessary and is only performed if the dog is lame on the contralateral leg. Lameness often resolves, presumably because the dog takes excessive

141

weight on this leg when the first shoulder is operated on and this results in early detachment of the cartilaginous flap and relief from pain (see page 139).

Complications
1   Excessive muscle damage during exposure and possibly failure to close the joint capsule may lead to seroma formation within a few days of surgery. The content of the seroma is aspirated with a needle as necessary.
2   Skin overlying the shoulder is very mobile, wound healing may be slower than normal and skin sutures are left *in situ* for at least 10 days to avoid the risk of wound breakdown.

Osteosarcoma

The proximal humerus is a common site for osteosarcoma in older dogs (see p. 23).

Fractures of the humerus

The majority of fractures of the humerus with the exception of condylar fractures, are caused in road traffic accidents. As a general rule, humeral fractures are treated by internal fixation because it is difficult to satisfy the main criteria for using external fixation, in particular the immobilization of the joint above and below the fracture. Chest injuries, particularly pneumothorax, are common complications of humeral fractures. Other possibilities include intrapulmonary haemorrhage, diaphragmatic rupture, rib fractures and occasionally chylothorax. A careful clinical and radiological examination should be done to check for and, if necessary, treat chest injuries before embarking on fracture fixation. Cases with closed pneumothorax or intrapulmonary haemorrhage are an anaesthetic risk and surgery should be delayed, (usually a matter of several days), until resolution occurs. During this period the dog is kept strictly confined in a kennel and the fractured humerus is immobilized with a Thomas extension splint, Velpeau dressing or a body cast. Sometimes early fracture repair must be undertaken in a

142

dog with a pneumothorax, for example, the heavy animal with multiple limb bone fractures. Under these circumstances the pneumothorax can be relieved with a chest drain which is inserted before anaesthesia is induced.

The majority of humeral shaft fractures follow the curvature of the musculospiral groove and are spiral or oblique in nature. The radial nerve lies close to the fracture site and paralysis is a common complication. Fortunately the paralysis is invariably transient and resolves within 2–3 weeks of fracture repair. Nevertheless, the nerve should be inspected during open reduction of shaft fractures and carefully protected during insertion of implants. Fractures of the humerus can be broadly classified (Braden 1975) into three groups:

1   Fractures involving the proximal epiphysis and metaphysis.
2   Fractures of the shaft.
3   Distal humeral fractures (supracondylar, condylar and intercondylar fractures).

The approximate distribution of fractures between these three groups has been quoted as 3%, 40% and 52% (Braden 1975). Methods of repair of humeral fractures have been described (Brinker 1974; Braden 1975).

Fractures of the humeral shaft

The medullary cavity of the humerus is wide proximally and gradually decreases in size towards the supratrochlear foramen. Consequently, although fractures do occur in the proximal shaft the majority involve the distal two–thirds and in particular the distal third. Fractures of the proximal and mid–shaft regions tend to be transverse while the more distal fractures follow the curvature of the musculospiral groove and are spiral or oblique in nature. Many are also comminuted.

Methods of fixation

INTRAMEDULLARY PIN
Although an intramedullary pin can be used for fixation of

143

shaft fractures of the humerus, rotational stability is usually poor because of the shape of the medullary cavity which is wide proximally and narrow distally. The method should be reserved for small breeds of dog which have transverse fractures which will impact under weight bearing. Pre-operatively, radiographs are taken of both the fractured humerus and the normal humerus. The normal is used as a guide to select a pin of the correct diameter to fit the medullary cavity as snuggly as possible. If necessary, the length of pin required can be assessed at this stage. The pin is partially transected with a hacksaw; the surgeon is then able to break it off flush with the surface of the greater tuberosity after insertion. The position of the fracture influences the length and diameter of pin required. For fractures involving the proximal or mid–shaft region, the pin is driven down the shaft to a point just proximal to the supratrachlear foramen (Fig. 171a). For fractures involving the distal third, a smaller diameter pin is used. The pin should be directed towards the medial side of the shaft so that the tip bypasses the supratrachlear foramen and is embedded in the medial condyle (Fig. 171b). A standard

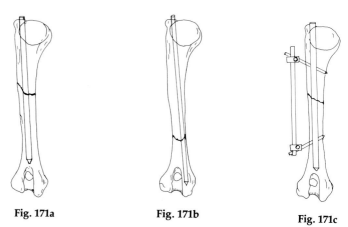

Fig. 171a   Fig. 171b

                                              Fig. 171c

anterolateral approach p. 147 is used to expose the humeral shaft and fracture site. The method of insertion of the pin is a matter of personal preference, but the author prefers retrograde pinning. The pin is driven up the shaft from the fracture site, keeping the shoulder flexed and the pin

144

directed towards the lateral side of the greater tuberosity. Once the tip of the pin has emerged, it is grasped with the Jacob's chuck and drawn up the shaft sufficiently to permit reduction of the fracture. Reduction of the fracture is maintained with bone holding forceps while the pin is driven into the distal shaft. When it has been inserted to the correct depth the pin is broken off flush with the bone (or cut with a saw or pin cutters). To minimize the risk of rotation and subsequent non–union, a body cast is applied for 3–4 weeks post operatively (Fig. 34a). Alternatively a ½ Kirschner device can be used to supplement the intra-medullary pin (Fig. 171c).

Lag screws
Lag screws can be used for internal fixation of oblique or spiral fractures of the humerus in small dogs when the length of the fracture is 4 times the diameter of the shaft (Fig. 172). However, external support with a body cast should also be provided.

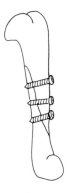

Fig. 172

Plate fixation
Plate fixation is the preferred method of treatment for fractures of the humeral shaft. Ideally the plate should be placed on the anterior aspect of the bone, this is the tensile side (see page 57). However the plate may also be placed on the lateral or medial side of the bone. Choice of site is dependent on the type of fracture and its position. Lag

145

screws are used for the initial fixation of oblique or comminuted fractures and the position of these screws in relation to the plate must be considered in the choice of approach. Figs. 173–188 illustrate some typical fractures of the humeral shaft with surgical approach and mode of fixation.

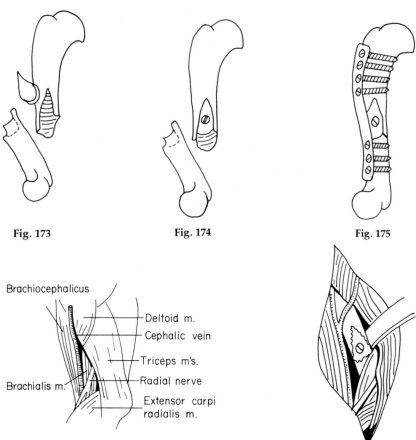

Fig. 173

Fig. 174

Fig. 175

Brachiocephalicus

Deltoid m.
Cephalic vein
Triceps m's.
Radial nerve
Extensor carpi radialis m.

Brachialis m.

Fig. 176

Fig. 177

The prognosis following plate fixation of humeral shaft fractures is generally good, but fracture reduction and insertion of the implants, especially in comminuted fractures is not easy. The chances of a successful outcome may be jeopardized through wound infection and osteomyelitis when operating time is prolonged. The likelihood of this

146

complication is minimized by strict asepsis, antibiotic prophylaxis and by keeping surgery time to a minimum. The inexperienced surgeon will be wise to refer comminuted shaft fractures of the humerus to a specialist for treatment.

A COMMINUTED MID-SHIFT FRACTURE OF THE HUMERUS

A lateral view is shown in Fig. 173. Fig. 174 shows how the butterfly fragment is reduced and fixation achieved with a lag screw; finally (Fig. 175) the plate is contoured and applied to the anterior aspect of the humerus.

An anterolateral approach is used to expose this fracture. A skin incision is made from the greater tuberosity to the lateral condyle. The cephalic vein is identified. The brachiocephalicus and brachialis muscles are separated and retracted to expose the shaft of the humerus (Fig. 176). The radial nerve is easily identified by separating the brachialis from the lateral head of the triceps. The nerve can then be traced distally as it runs around the brachialis to emerge on its lateral aspect at the level of the extensor carpi radialis muscle (Fig. 176).

In exposure of the distal anterior surface of the shaft the brachialis is retracted laterally and used to protect the radial nerve (Fig. 177). The proximal surface of the humerus is exposed by subperiosteal elevation between the pectoral and deltoid muscles.

A COMMINUTED FRACTURE INVOLVING THE DISTAL THIRD OF THE HUMERUS

A lateral view of the fracture appears in Fig. 178. In Fig. 179 the butterfly fragment has been reduced and fixation achieved with 2 lag screws. Figs. 180 and 181 show how the plate is contoured and applied to the lateral aspect of the humerus (* indicates lag screws).

The antero-lateral approach is used to expose the fracture (Figs. 176 and 177). In addition, the brachialis muscle and radial nerve are mobilized so that the plate can be slid beneath them on the lateral aspect of the humerus (Fig. 182). The origin of the extensor carpi radialis muscle is freed from the lateral condyle to complete exposure of the distal humerus.

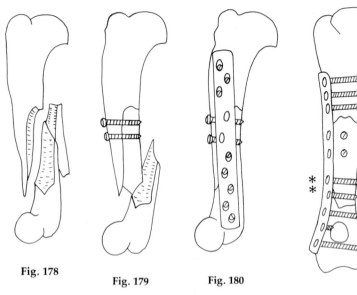

Fig. 178

Fig. 179

Fig. 180

Fig. 181

A lateral view of the fracture is shown in Fig. 183. Initial fixation is by interfragmentary compression using 2 lag screws (Fig. 184). Then the plate is contoured and applied to the medial side of the humerus (Figs. 185, 186).

A skin incision is made over the medial aspect of the humerus. The median nerve and the biceps muscle are retracted cranially and the ulnar nerve and medial head of the triceps caudally to expose the humeral shaft. Branches of the brachial artery and vein run with the nerves and should be protected. The medial side of the humerus is relatively flat and is an ideal surface for the application of a plate. However, exposure of the humerus is limited proximally by the pectoral muscles and the brachial blood vessels (Fig. 187).

SUPRACONDYLAR FRACTURES OF THE HUMERUS

In supracondylar fractures, the fracture line passes through the supratrochlear foramen. The fractures tend to be transverse or oblique in nature and some are also comminuted.

148

In immature dogs, the fracture may take the form of a Salter Type II epiphyseal separation.

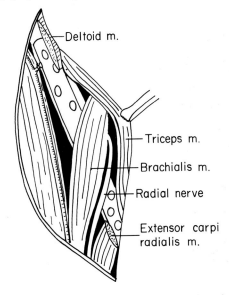

—Deltoid m.

—Triceps m.

—Brachialis m.

—Radial nerve

—Extensor carpi radialis m.

Fig. 182

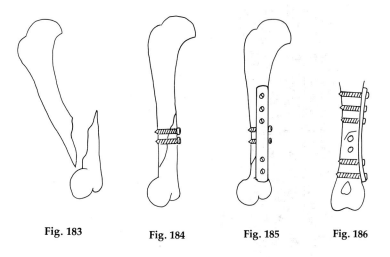

Fig. 183   **Fig. 184**   **Fig. 185**   **Fig. 186**

Supracondylar fractures must be accurately reduced and rigidly stabilized because of their proximity to the elbow joint.

149

A medial approach is used to expose the fracture (see page 148). There are several ways of stabilizing the fracture. One of the simplest (Brinker 1974) is to use an intra-medullary pin (retrograde introduction page 144) which is driven down the shaft into the medial condyle. Rotation is prevented with a Kirschner wire placed obliquely across the fracture site from the lateral condyle (Fig. 188).

Rush pins introduced through each of the humeral condyles into the humeral shaft (Fig. 189) also provides a satisfactory method of treating supracondylar fractures.

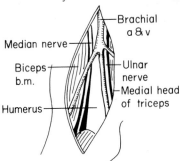

Fig. 187

At this clinic three other methods are frequently used. In oblique supracondylar fractures or oblique fractures extending through the distal humeral growth plate, 2 lag screws are used for fixation (Fig. 190). The first screw is placed transversely just proximal to the supra trochlear foramen and the second screw is driven up through the medial condyle. In immature dogs the screws are removed as soon as healing is complete (approximately 4 weeks) to prevent premature closure of the growth plate.

Transverse supracondylar fractures can be stabilized with a single lag screw introduced through the medial condyle, but further support should be given with a body case for 3 weeks following surgery (Fig. 34a).

In large dogs, especially those with comminuted supracondylar fractures, a plate is applied to the medial side of the humerus. For adequate stability 2 screws should be placed in the distal fragment (Fig. 191). If there is only room for one then additional support with a body cast should be given for 3 weeks following surgery. Braden (1975) recommends a caudal approach for comminuted supracondylar

150

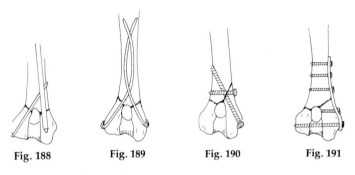

Fig. 188   Fig. 189   Fig. 190   Fig. 191

fractures in large dogs (see p. 157) with the application of two plates on the posterior aspect of the supratrochlear ridges. This method of fixation is described in more detail under the management of 'T' and 'Y' fractures of the humerus (see p. 157).

Condylar fractures of the humerus

The management of condylar fractures described here is based on a series of 133 cases treated by the author (Denny 1983). There are areas of structural weakness in the distal humerus which predispose to certain types of fracture (Shuttleworth 1938; Walker & Hickman 1958). The humeral trochlea (Fig. 192) is separated from the shaft by the

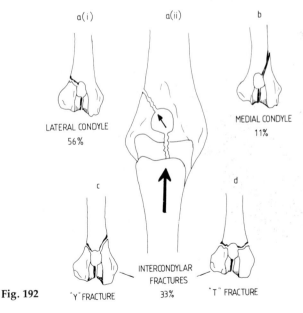

Fig. 192

a(i)

LATERAL CONDYLE
56%

a(ii)

b

MEDIAL CONDYLE
11%

c

'Y' FRACTURE

INTERCONDYLAR
FRACTURES
33%

d

'T' FRACTURE

supratrochlear foramen. Main support for the trochlea is provided by the medial epicondyle which is in effect a direct extension of the humeral shaft. Laterally, the trochlea is supported by the lateral epicondyle but this is a far weaker structure than its medial counterpart. Condylar fractures usually result from a violent upward stress transmitted through the head of the radius onto the humeral trochlea, for example, when a dog falls or jumps from a height, taking excessive weight on the leg (Walker & Hickman 1958). It comes as no surprise that the lateral condyle which has the weakest attachments to the humeral shaft fractures most frequently (56% of cases). In the face of even greater stress, the medial condyle is also sheared from its attachments to the main shaft, giving rise to the intercondylar ('Y' or 'T') fracture (Fig. 192c,d). Intercondylar fractures occurred in 33% of cases; the fracture is referred to as a 'Y' fracture (Fig. 192c) if the supracondylar ridges are fractured obliquely, and 'T' fractures if the ridges are fractured transversely. Solitary fractures of the medial condyle occur in 11% of cases.

Condylar fractures, as with any intra–articular fracture, require accurate anatomical reduction and rigid internal fixation to promote primary bone union if normal joint function is to be restored. Basic methods of fixation were described by Knight (1956, 1959), and Walker & Hickman (1958); a variety of techniques were subsequently proposed (Brinker, 1974) and these have been reviewed by Braden (1975) and more recently by Payne–Johnson & Lewis (1981) and Denny (1983).

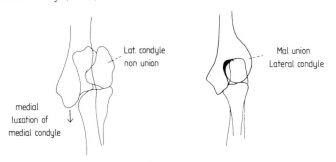

Fig. 193a   Fig. 193b

152

The commonest cause of fracture of the lateral condyle is a fall. The fracture occurs most often in dogs under a year of age (67% of cases) and the peak age incidence is at 4 months. The fracture is stabilized with a single lag screw driven through the lateral condyle into the medial condyle (Fig. 197b,c). Failure to treat the fracture surgically results in medial luxation of the medial condyle, because lateral support for the joint is lost. Malunion or non–union of the lateral condyle causes permanent joint deformity (Fig. 193a,b). The range of elbow movement remains limited and varying degrees of lameness persist. The prognosis is obviously better in immature dogs because of their ability to remodel the distal humerus following fracture.

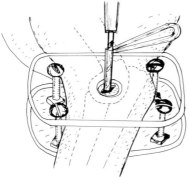

Fig. 194 Condyle clamp (constructed from 2 sheets of perspex+4 bolts), used to maintain reduction of a fractured lateral condyle. This allows a transcondylar lag screw to be inserted through a stab incision.

LAG SCREW FIXATION (Brinker 1979)
If the fracture of the lateral condyle is less than 12 hours old, there is usually little swelling and the unstable condyle can be easily palpated. Having prepared the leg for surgery the most prominent point of the lateral and medial condyle are grasped between finger and thumb and pressure is exerted while the elbow is extended; initially crepitus may be felt but if reduction is successful the lateral condyle will be felt to slip or click back into its normal position where it is maintained by thumb pressure. The elbow is maintained in the extended position and a condyle clamp (Fig. 194) is carefully slid into position. The holes of the clamp fit over the most

prominent points of the condyles and the clamp is tightened to maintain reduction. A check X–ray is taken; if reduction is satisfactory the leg is re–prepared for surgery and a transcondylar lag screw inserted through a stab incision made over the lateral condyle (details of correct positioning of the screw hole are given below).

If the fracture is more than 24 hours old considerable soft tissue swelling will have occurred and accurate closed reduction may be difficult as a result. Under these circumstances open reduction should be performed. A skin incision is made directly over the lateral condyle (Fig. 195a). The lateral head of the triceps muscle is exposed and the deep fascia along its anterior border incised (Fig. 195b). The muscle is retracted to expose the condyle (Fig. 195c). The

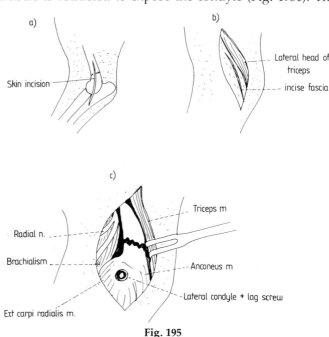

Fig. 195

radial nerve emerges between the lateral head of the triceps and the brachialis just proximal to the incision, but provided dissection is limited to the soft tissues directly over the lateral condyle and its supracondylar ridge there should be little risk of nerve damage during exposure. Haematoma or granulation tissue is removed from the intercondylar frac-

154

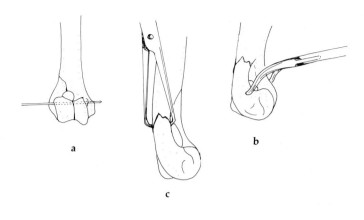

Fig. 196

ture site, the adjacent surfaces of the fractured supra-condylar ridge are cleaned of all soft tissue and reduction of the condyle can then be readily achieved by manipulation. If the fracture of the supracondylar ridge is accurately reduced it can be assumed that reduction of the intercondylar fracture site is also adequate. Temporary fixation is achieved with a transcondylar Kirschner wire (Fig. 196a). The wire is removed after insertion of the lag screw.

Alternatively, reduction can be maintained in the following ways:

1   By the application of Vulsellum forceps or ASIF reduction forceps to the condyles (Fig. 196b).

2   In small dogs the fractured supracondylar ridge can be stabilized with Allis tissue forceps (Fig. 196c).

3   In large dogs a Kirschner wire can be placed across the fractured supracondylar ridge.

The drill hole for the transcondylar lag screw is commenced immediately below and just in front of the most prominent point of the lateral condyle and directed to emerge at the corresponding spot on the medial condyle (Fig. 197a(i),a(ii)). If a cancellous screw is used for fixation, the threaded portion of the screw must grip entirely in the medial condyle (Fig. 197c). If a cortex screw is used then the

155

hole in the lateral condyle must be overdrilled to the same diameter as the screw to ensure that the lag effect is achieved as the screw is tightened giving compression of the fracture site (Figs 197a(ii), 197b).

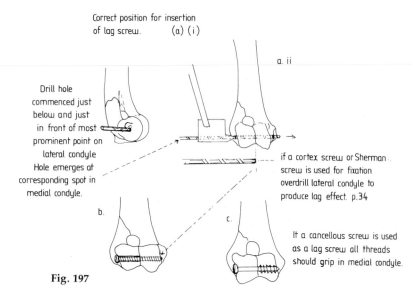

Correct position for insertion of lag screw. (a) (i)

a. ii

Drill hole commenced just below and just in front of most prominent point on lateral condyle. Hole emerges at corresponding spot in medial condyle.

if a cortex screw or Sherman screw is used for fixation overdrill lateral condyle to produce lag effect. p.34

b.

c.

It a cancellous screw is used as a lag screw all threads should grip in medial condyle.

Fig. 197

Lateral condylar fractures, provided they are adequately reduced and stabilized carry a good prognosis and the screw can be left *in situ*. The average recovery period is four weeks (range 2–8 weeks). 77% of dogs regain full limb function and 23% have slight or occasional lameness (Denny 1983).

FRACTURES OF THE MEDIAL CONDYLE

The commonest cause of fracture of the medial condyle is a fall and there is no specific age incidence for the injury. The same principles of treatment apply as for lateral condylar fractures, however the medial condylar fragment is often large enough to accept two lag screws, one transcondylar and one placed proximal to the supratrochlear foramen (Fig. 197d,e). Exposure of the medial condyle is described on page 148). Medial condylar fractures carry a similar prognosis to fractures of the lateral condyle.

156

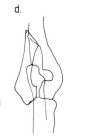
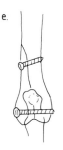

d.

e.

Tracing Pre and Post operative radiography
of a pointer with a fracture of the
medial condyle.

INTERCONDYLAR FRACTURES OF THE HUMERUS

Intercondylar, 'Y' or 'T' fractures are caused by falls or road
traffic accidents in most cases. There is no specific age
incidence. Treatment of these fractures is difficult and can
present a real challenge even to the most experienced of
orthopaedic surgeons. To permit adequate exposure and
accurate anatomical reduction of the fracture a caudal
approach to the elbow is recommended. (Figs. 198a–c). The
dog is placed in dorsal recumbency for surgery with the
affected leg pulled forward. A skin incision is made over the
caudolateral aspect of the elbow, the subcutaneous fat and

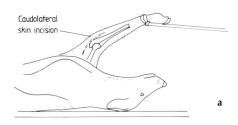

Caudolateral
skin incision

a

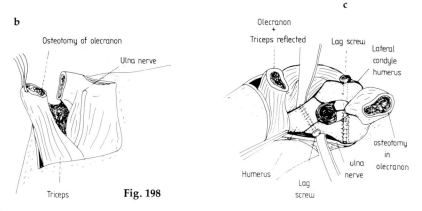

c

b

Osteotomy of olecranon

Ulna nerve

Olecranon
+
Triceps reflected

Lag screw

Lateral
condyle
humerus

osteotomy
in
olecranon

Humerus

ulna
nerve

Lag
screw

Triceps

Fig. 198

157

fascia are incised and undermined to allow reflection of skin from both sides of the elbow. Fascia along the cranial border of the medial head of the triceps is incised and the ulna nerve is identified and retracted (Fig. 198b) from the olecranon. The anterior margin of the lateral head of the triceps is also freed from fascial attachments. Transverse osteotomy of the olecranon is performed with an oscillating saw, or hack saw, distal to the tendon of insertion of the triceps on the olecranon and proximal to the anconeal process (Fig. 198b). (After repair of the intercondylar fracture the olecranon is re–attached using Kirschner wires or a screw in combination with a wire tension band (see Fig. 219a)). (If a screw is used the screw hole should be prepared before the osteotomy of the olecranon is performed).

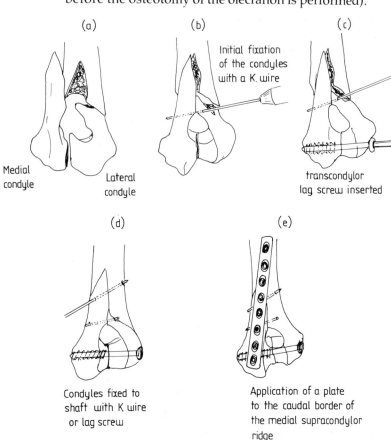

(a)

Medial condyle

Lateral condyle

(b)

Initial fixation of the condyles with a K. wire

(c)

transcondylar lag screw inserted

(d)

Condyles fixed to shaft with K wire or lag screw

(e)

Application of a plate to the caudal border of the medial supracondylar ridge

Fig. 199

158

The olecranon is reflected with the attached triceps muscle mass and remnants of the anconeus muscle are reflected as necessary to complete exposure (Fig. 198c) of the entire caudal surface of the elbow joint. The condyles are reduced first. The easiest way of doing this is to reduce the proximal ends of the condyles and fix them with a Kirschner wire in a 'T' fracture or lag screw in a 'Y' fracture (Fig. 199b). Then complete reduction of the articular surface of the condyles and insert a transcondylar lag screw (Fig. 199c). Generally the screw is inserted from lateral to medial. The humeral condyles are attached to the shaft of the humerus with a Kirschner wire or lag screw (Fig. 199d), then a plate is applied to the posterior aspect of the medial supracondylar ridge (Fig. 199e). In large dogs a second smaller plate can be applied to the lateral supracondylar ridge (Braden 1975).

The olecranon osteotomy is repaired as described above and subsequent wound closure is routine. A Robert Jones Bandage is applied for a week post–operatively to provide support and control post–operative swelling.

Intercondylar fractures carry a moderate prognosis, 46% of dogs regain normal limb function, 36% have slight or occasional lameness and 18% have moderate to severe lameness as a result of deformity and osteoarthritis. (Denny 1983).

THE ELBOW JOINT

The elbow is a ginglymus joint. The ligaments of the joint are illustrated in Figs. 200 and 201. Soft tissue structures of surgical importance are shown in the surgical approaches to the elbow.

Developmental disorders of the elbow can be summarized as follows:

1   Ununited anconeal process (Fig. 202, 1).
2   Osteochondritis dissecans of the medial condyle of the humerus (Fig. 202, 2).
3   Ununited coronoid process (Fig. 202, 3).
4   Congenital dislocation of the elbow.
5   Caudal subluxation of the elbow following premature closure of the distal ulnar epiphyseal plate.

159

6 Premature closure of the distal radial epiphyseal plate resulting in a short radius and elbow instability.

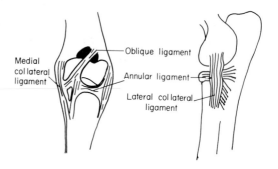

Fig. 200. Elbow, cranial view.   **Fig. 201.** Elbow, lateral view.

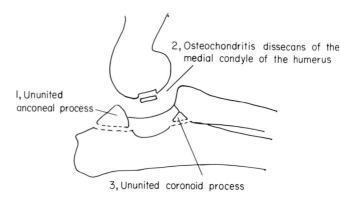

Fig. 202

Figs. 200 & 201 reproduced by permission of Miller M.E. (1952). *A Guide to the Dissection of the Dog.* 3rd. Ed. Edwards Brothers. Michigan.

Ununited Anconeal Process (Van Sickle 1966; Ljunggren *et al* 1966; Bradney 1967; Corley *et al* 1968; Hanlon 1969)

Ununited anconeal process is a well recognised problem in the Alsatian and the Basset Hound. The condition occasionally occurs in other large breeds. In affected animals the anconeal process develops as a separate ossification centre. The process should unite with the olecranon by the time the dog is 5 months old. Non union results in elbow instability and osteoarthrosis.

160

Affected animals present with a gradual onset of lameness, at 4 to 5 months of age. There is pain on palpation of the elbow, particularly when it is forcibly extended. There may be obvious crepitus and in longstanding cases, the elbow becomes thickened and the range of joint movement is limited due to osteoarthrosis. A flexed lateral radiograph of the elbow will confirm the diagnosis (Fig. 203). The condition is bilateral in 40% of cases, consequently both elbows should be radiographed.

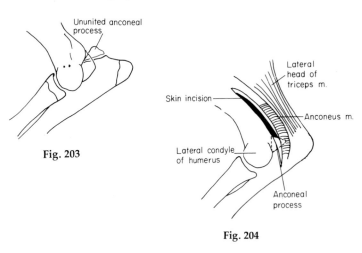

Fig. 203

Fig. 204

Treatment is by surgical excision of the anconeal process. A skin incision is made along the posterolateral border of the humerus (Fig. 204). The cranial edge of the lateral head of the triceps is retracted caudally to expose the anconeus muscle. The anconeus muscle together with the joint capsule to which it is closely attached are incised just caudal to the lateral condyle (leaving sufficient muscle on the condylar side to be sutured). Haemorrhage from the muscle may be a problem but this can be controlled by using self-retaining retractors to retract the muscle edges and expose the caudal aspect of the elbow joint. The elbow is flexed to reveal the anconeal process which is prised away from its cartilagious attachments to the ulna with a periosteal elevator. After removal of the process, the joint is flushed out with normal saline and the anconeus muscle and joint capsule closed together with a continuous catgut suture. Subsequent wound closure is routine. A support bandage is applied for a week post-operatively and exercise is restricted for 4 weeks. If the lesion is bilateral, a 6-week interval is left between operations.

The anconeal process normally contributes to the stability of the elbow joint. Instability after removal may predispose the dog to intermittent elbow sprains and osteoarthrosis. Grøndalen and Rørkvik (1980), in a follow up of 37 dogs treated for ununited anconeal process, reported that 39% of the cases were occasionally lame after exercise or were stiff after rest.

It might be expected that the dislocation of the elbow is more likely to occur after removal of the anconeal process. This does not occur, presumably because scar formation after surgery provides sufficient stability.

Osteochondritis Dissecans of the Medial Condyle of the Humerus (Olsson 1975; Wood *et al* 1975; McCurnin *et al* 1976; Leighton 1978; Denny & Gibbs 1980).

OCD of the medial condyle of the humerus is a common cause of elbow lameness in the Labrador, Retriever and Rottweiler. There is a gradual onset of lameness at 4–5 months of age. Lameness tends to be intermittent in nature and is often most obvious, either when the dog gets up from resting, or after exercise. There is pain on forced extension of the elbow and the degree of pain can be increased by supinating the forearm during extension. Elbow thickening may be appreciated especially in chronic cases.

Radiographic diagnosis is not easy especially in the early stages. A flexed later view, an AP view and in some cases an oblique AP view should be taken of both elbows. OCD rapidly causes osteoarthrosis in the elbow. The first indication of this is osteophyte formation on the caudal aspect of the anconeal process (Fig. 205b), giving it a 'fuzzy' appearance. Later similar changes develop on the medial aspect of the elbow (Fig. 205a) and on the head of the radius (Fig. 205b). The AP view of the elbow may demonstrate the OCD lesion as a small erosion in the subchondral bone of the medial condyle of the humerus (Fig. 205a). However, this feature cannot be demonstrated in every case of osteochondritis dissecans.

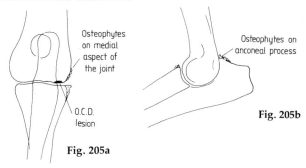

Osteophytes on medial aspect of the joint

O.C.D. lesion

Fig. 205a

Osteophytes on anconeal process

Fig. 205b

Surgical treatment should be undertaken early to prevent the development of osteoarthrosis. There is little to be gained by surgery once joint changes have become advanced.

Ununited coronoid process (Olsson 1975; McCurnin *et al* 1876; Denny & Gibbs 1980)

Failure of the coronoid process to unite with the ulna is an osteochondritis–type lesion of the elbow. The condition affects the Labrador, Retriever and Rottweiler and occasionally dogs have both OCD and ununited coronoid process in the same joint. The history and clinical signs associated with ununited coronoid process are identical to osteochondritis dissecans. Ununited coronoid process also causes the rapid development of osteoarthrosis with a similar distribution of osteophytes as described under OCD. An oblique AP view of the elbow may demonstrate the ununited coronoid process (Fig. 206) but even in positive cases the radiographic findings may not be conclusive. Nevertheless, if a Labrador, Retriever or Rottweiler under a year oaf age is presented with chronic foreleg lameness, pain can be localised to the elbow and there is radiographic evidence of osteoarthrosis, then an exploratory medial arthrotomy is justified. The medial approach gives access to both OCD lesions and ununited coronoid process.

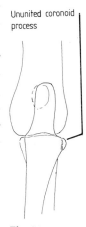

Ununited coronoid process

Fig. 206

Elbow–medial arthrotomy technique

After routine surgical preparation, the dog is placed on its side and a bolster is placed beneath the elbow (Fig. 207a). A skin incision is made over the medial humeral condyle (Fig. 207a). The Pronator teres and flexor carpi radialis muscles are separated close to their origin on the medial epicondyle and retracted with a West's retractor (Arnold Vet Products Ltd). A vertical incision is made into the joint capsule over the humeral condyle only (Fig. 207b). The blades of a pair of straight scissors are then introduced between the articular surfaces of the joint and spread laterally to complete exposure (Fig. 207c). The West's retractor is repositioned to include the cut edges of the joint capsule. This method of arthrotomy minimizes the risk of damage to the median

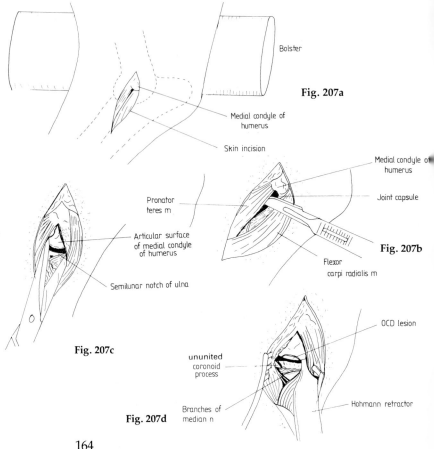

Bolster

Fig. 207a

Medial condyle of humerus

Skin incision

Medial condyle of humerus

Joint capsule

Pronator teres m

Articular surface of medial condyle of humerus

Fig. 207b

Flexor carpi radialis m

Semilunar notch of ulna

Fig. 207c

OCD lesion

ununited coronoid process

Hohmann retractor

Branches of median n

Fig. 207d

164

nerve and artery which cross the anterior and distal margins of the joint. The articular surfaces are separated with the aid of Hohmann retractors and exposure is improved with the aid of an assistant who exerts pressure on the forearm and 'hinges' the elbow over the bolster (Fig. 207d).

The medial condyle of the humerus (Fig. 207d) is inspected for an osteochondritis dissecans lesion. If a cartilaginous flap is present, it is removed and the underlying erosion in the subchondral bone is curetted. In some cases the lesion takes the form of fissures in the cartilage; this area is curetted. If there is no evidence of osteochondritis dissecans the coronoid process is inspected, freed from any remaining cartilaginous or fibrous attachments and removed. The coronoid process will be found either as a discrete triangular fragment of bone and cartilage or it may be in the form of two or three fragments. The coronoid process lies immediately beneath the medial collateral ligament and exposure can be improved by cutting the caudal margin of the collateral ligament, however complete section of the ligament should not be necessary.

Osteochondritis dissecans and ununited coronoid process have the same aetiology (Olsson 1975) and consequently it is wise to inspect the coronoid process even when there is an obvious osteochondritis dissecans lesion present as both conditions can co–exist. After the lesion has been dealt with, the joint is flushed out with saline. The muscle bellies are coated with continuous suture of catgut which effectively seals the joint capsule. The rest of the wound closure is carried out in routine fashion.

Post operative care
The elbow is supported with a bandage for one week. Antibiotic cover is given for 5 days and skin sutures are removed at 7 days. Exercise is restricted for 4 weeks and then gradually increased. In dogs with bilateral lesions, a 6 week interval is left between operations. Normal limb function is generally regained within 2 months of surgery and subsequent follow up reveals little increase in the degree of osteoarthritis present at the time of surgery (Denny & Gibbs 1980).

Complications

Osteoarthrosis present at the time of surgery or secondary to surgical interference may lead to poor exercise tolerance with varying degrees of lameness and a limited range of elbow movement.

Surgical exposure of the osteochondritis dissecans lesion or ununited coronoid process in the elbow can be difficult for the inexperienced surgeon and failure to identify and treat either lesion will result in progressive osteoarthrosis.

Ununited medial epicondyle (Vaughan 1979; Denny 1983)

Failure of the medial epicondyle to unite with the humerus is occasionally encountered as a fusion defect in immature Labradors. History and clinical signs are similar to osteo-chondritis dissecans of the elbow. Radiographic examination shows the ununited epicondyle as a discrete fragment on the medial side of the elbow (Fig. 208a). There are numerous muscle attachments to the fragment. If it is large, then it should be reattached to the humerus with a lag screw (Fig. 208b). If the fragment is small, lameness will generally resolve by the time the dog reaches 1 year of age.

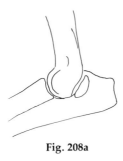

Fig. 208a

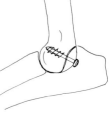

Fig. 208b

Congenital dislocation of the elbow

Congenital dislocation of the elbow is seen in small breeds of dog, particularly the Pekingese. Larger breeds such as the Staffordshire Bull Terrier, Labrador and Mastiff are also

166

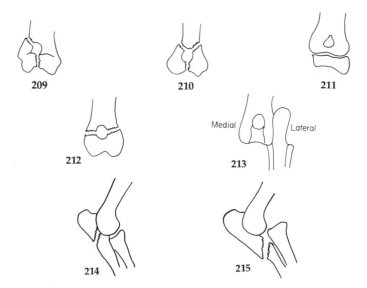

209

210

211

Medial   Lateral

212

213

214

215

Fig. 209. Fracture of the lateral or medial condyle. Fig. 210. 'Y' fracture. Fig. 211. Distal epiphyseal separation. Fig. 212. Supracondylar fracture. Fig. 213. Dislocation of the elbow. Fig. 214. Fracture of the olecranon. Fig. 215. Fracture of the ulna with anterior dislocation of the radial head.

occasionally affected. There is usually lateral luxation of the radial head; this can be detected on palpation and the range of elbow movement is limited. An AP radiograph of the joint will confirm the diagnosis. The condition is often bilateral. Affected animals are not greatly incapacitated by the deformity and no treatment is needed, except restricted exercise until the dog reaches 1 year of age.

Subluxation of the elbow following growth disturbances of the radius and ulna

These conditions are described on pages 174, 177.

Traumatic conditions of the elbow (Figs. 209–215)

Dislocation of the elbow joint

Dislocation of the elbow is seen in dogs over a year of age. The injury is caused in road traffic accidents or when a dog catches its leg in a fence and is suspended by the limb..

The radial head dislocates laterally and this can only occur if the anconeal process has become disengaged from its fossa between the humeral condyles. Therefore the elbow must be flexed by more than 45° in the accident and twisted for dislocation to occur, and provided this concept is grasped then a rational method of reduction can be employed (see below).

After dislocation of the elbow the affected limb is held forward, abducted and supinated. The elbow joint is painful and flexion and extension are limited.

Reduction is achieved under general anaesthesia by fully flexing the elbow, the radius and ulna are then rotated medially and the elbow joint is slowly extended until the anconeal process is re-engaged in its normal position between the humeral condyles.

If the manipulation is successful the radial head and anconeal process 'snap' back into place, a full range of elbow movement is restored and the joint should feel stable.

No further treatment should be necessary except to apply a support bandage for a week and restrict exercise for four weeks.

Occasionally the elbow remains unstable due to stretching or rupture of the collateral ligaments. Stability can be restored by replacing the medial collateral ligament with a wire prosthesis anchored by two screws, one placed in the medial condyle of the humerus and the other in the ulna (Fig. 216).

In longstanding neglected dislocations open reduction must be carried out but this can be difficult. The operation is done in two stages. First reduction is achieved through a lateral approach to the elbow, fibrous adhesions are broken down and the radial head and anconeal process are levered back into their normal position with a periosteal elevator inserted into the joint space. The lateral wound is closed, the dog turned over and the medial aspect of the joint exposed. A wire medial collateral ligament prosthesis is inserted as in Fig. 216 to prevent redislocation.

The prosthesis is not removed unless the screws loosen or eventual fracture of the wire leads to soft tissue reaction.

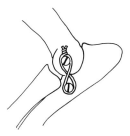

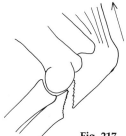

Fig. 217

Fig. 216

Fracture of the olecranon

Fracture of the olecranon is illustrated in Fig. 217, the fragment is distracted by the strong pull of the triceps tendon and this can only be overcome by internal fixation. Most fractures occur through the semilunar notch, the articular margin of the fracture serves as a fulcrum and if an intramedullary pin or a screw is used for fixation as in Fig. 218 it

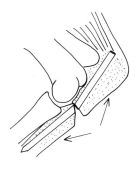

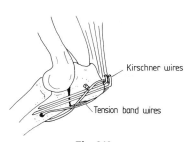

Kirschner wires

Tension band wires

Fig. 219a

Fig. 218

will be subjected to excessive bending forces and will often break before fracture healing is complete unless the elbow is immobilized in a plaster cast. This problem can be overcome and the tensile forces of the triceps used to advantage to compress the fracture by using the wire tension band for fixation, see Fig. 219a. Alternatively, a plate can be used for fixation and this method is indicated for comminuted fractures of the olecranon. The plate is applied to the lateral aspect of the ulna (Fig. 219b).

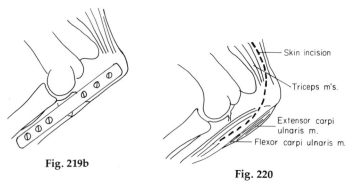

Skin incision

Triceps m's.

Extensor carpi ulnaris m.

Flexor carpi ulnaris m.

Fig. 219b

Fig. 220

Exposure of the olecranon is achieved through a curved caudolateral skin incision, the extensor carpi ulnaris muscle and the flexor carpi ulnaris muscle are separated and retracted to reveal the shaft of the ulna (Fig. 220).

Fractures of the radial head

Fractures of the radial head are rare. Management of these fractures has been described by Neal (1975). Open reduction is indicated to restore the integrity of the joint surface and fixation is achieved with a lag screw or Kirschner wire depending on the size of the fragment. If the fracture is comminuted and cannot be stabilized, then excision of the radial head can be performed as a salvage procedure.

Monteggia fracture

Fracture of the ulna with anterior dislocation of the radial

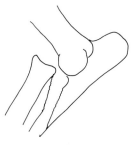

Fig. 221

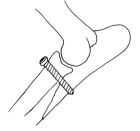

Fig. 222

head is commonly called a 'Monteggia fracture', after the condition in man (Boyd and Boals 1969). The injury is rare and only 5 cases have been seen at his clinic during a 10 year period.

Anterior dislocation of the radial head occurs when the annular ligament which normally binds the radial head to the proximal ulna ruptures and the ulna fractures just distal to the elbow. The ulna shaft is firmly attached to the radius by the interosseous ligament and consequently moves with it in an anterior direction (Fig. 221).

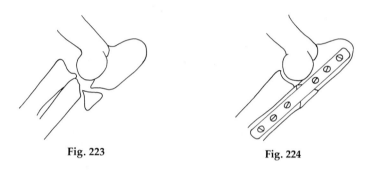

Fig. 223   Fig. 224

Provided the injury is recent, the dislocation of the radial head can be easily reduced by manipulation and because of the strong interosseous attachment between the radius and ulna reduction can be maintained by the repair of the ulna fracture alone. This is done with a plate (Figs 223 & 224) or intramedullary pin and wire tension band. An alternative method is to place a lag screw through the head of the radius into the proximal ulna to restore stability (Fig. 222). Exposure of the head of the radius is described under the management of shaft fractures of the radius and ulna.

Arthrodesis of the elbow

Arthrodesis of the elbow is occasionally indicated when painful osteoarthritic change has occurred or when neoplasia or osteomyelitis involves the olecranon. The elbow is exposed through a caudolateral incision, the tendon of insertion of the triceps is severed and the olecranon resected through the semilunar notch. After removal of the olecranon the articular cartilage of the elbow is removed and the joint spaces packed with a cancellous bone graft. Fixation is achieved by the application of a plate to the caudal surface of the humerus and ulna (Fig. 225).

The main risk of arthrodesis of a major joint is that a longer lever arm is created and that even minor trauma can result in a long bone fracture, the radius and ulna being affected in the case of an elbow arthrodesis.

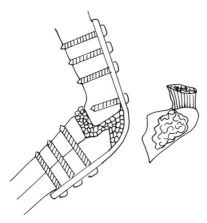

Fig. 225

Growth disturbances of the radius and ulna (Denny 1976)

Longitudinal growth of the radius and ulna occurs from the proximal and distal growth plates (Fig. 226). The distal growth plates contribute approximately 70% of the final length of the radius and 85% of the ulna (Parkes *et al* 1966). The remaining percentage is derived from the proximal growth plates, however in the ulna this plate contributes more to the length of the olecranon than to the shaft of the bone.

The radius and ulna lie parallel to each other and their rate of growth is closely inter-related. A growth disturbance occurs when there is a discrepancy in the rate of growth between two bones: this is caused by either premature closure or a decrease in the rate of growth at one growth plate while growth at the adjacent plate continues normally.

172

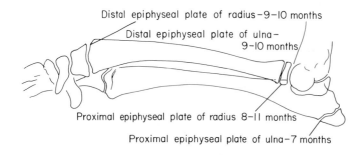

Distal epiphyseal plate of radius – 9–10 months

Distal epiphyseal plate of ulna – 9–10 months

Proximal epiphyseal plate of radius 8–11 months

Proximal epiphyseal plate of ulna – 7 months

Fig. 226

Growth disturbances of the radius and ulna caused by premature closure of the distal ulnar growth plate are seen most frequently in giant breeds of dog, especially Great Danes and Irish Wolfhounds. It is usually the largest pup in the litter that is affected and predisposing factors are over-feeding and uncontrolled exercise during puppyhood. Growth disturbances can also be precipitated by trauma. A serious potential complication of fracture of the distal third of the radius in puppies is premature closure of the distal ulnar growth plate and if untreated, severe limb deformity will result.

The degree and type of deformity seen depends on the age of the animal at the time of injury and the growth plate involved. The approximate times of closure of the epiphyses of the radius and ulna are given in Fig. 226. The radiological features of forelimb growth disturbances have been reviewed and described by O'Brien *et al* (1971).

PREMATURE CLOSURE OF THE DISTAL ULNAR GROWTH PLATE

Premature closure of the distal ulnar growth plate causes the following deformities. Growth of the radius continues at the normal rate, but the direction of growth is impeded by the 'bow-string' effect of the ulna; consequently there is firstly anterior and then medial bowing of the radius causing lateral deviation of the foot (Carpal valgus deformity). Later, external rotation of the carpus and sub-

173

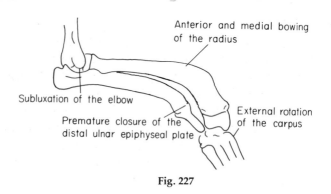

Fig. 227

luxation of the elbow occurs (Fig. 227) as the head of the
radius pushes the humeral condyles proximally.

With any growth deformity, radiographs should be taken
which include the elbow and carpal joints of both limbs for
comparison of the growth plates and assessment of the
degree of deformity and changes in the joints.

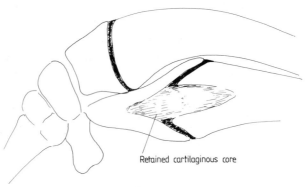

Fig. 228

In many Danes and Irish Wolfhounds presented with
lateral deviation of the carpus, radiographs show that the
ulnar growth plate is still open. The growth plate cartilage is
failing to ossify normally and appears as an elongated radiolucent zone. The zone is called a retained cartilaginous core
(Fig. 228) and it signifies that the ulna growth plate is
growing more slowly than its distal radial counterpart.

The average age of dogs presented with growth disturbances is 5 months and therefore it is necessary to consider

174

what can be done to prevent further deformity during the remaining period of growth. The use of plaster casts or splints to maintain alignment is usually unsuccessful.

If both distal radial and ulnar growth plates are *still open,* lateral deviation of the carpus can be corrected by placing a staple across the medial side of the distal radial growth plate (Fig. 230). This temporarily delays growth on the medial side of the leg while continued growth of the ulna and lateral side of the distal radial growth plate straightens the leg. The process usually takes 4–6 weeks.

TECHNIQUE FOR STAPLING THE MEDIAL SIDE OF THE DISTAL RADIAL GROWTH PLATE (Vaughan 1976)

1 The leg is prepared for surgery in routine fashion.

2 A 19 gauge needle is inserted into the medial side of the distal radial growth plate. The needle should slide easily into soft cartilage (Fig. 229).

3 AP and lateral radiographs are taken to check the position of the needle. The needle is then used as a landmark to decide the correct position for the staple.

4 The dog is taken into the operating theatre, the leg is repreped with hibitane and draped. A longitudinal incision is made directly over the growth plate (there is no need to incise the periosteum). The staple is pushed into the bone making sure that the bars of the stable are on either side of the growth plate as judged from the position of the guide needle on the radiographs (Fig. 230). The staple is driven

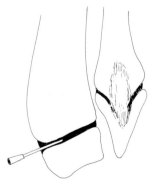

Fig. 229

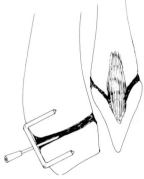

Fig. 230

into the bone with a hammer. The guide needle is removed and the skin is closed with horizontal mattress sutures. Check X–rays are taken to ensure that the staple is correctly placed and a support bandage is applied for 1 week. The leg generally takes 4–6 weeks to straighten. The staple must then be removed (unless the dog is almost fully grown) otherwise the carpus will tend to deviate medially. Exercise is restricted to short walks while the staple is *in situ*.

If the distal ulnar growth plate has closed prematurely then in addition to stapling the radius, a 1–2 cm section of the ulnar shaft must be removed to relieve the bow string effect and allow growth of the radius to continue un-impeded (Newton 1974) (Figs 231 and 232). The gap in the ulnar shaft regardless of size, rapidly fills with callus. (A 2 cm defect is bridged within 4–6 weeks). It is sometimes necessary to repeat the osteotomy before the dog is fully grown.

Ulnar osteotomy and stapling are designed to prevent further deformity and correct angulation of the radius in the

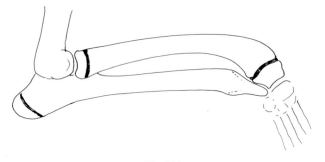

Fig. 231

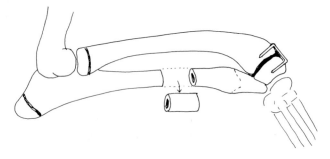

Fig. 232

growing dog after premature closure or retarded growth has occurred at the distal ulnar growth plate. Once the distal radial growth plate has closed then the only method of straightening the limb is by wedge osteotomy of the radius and ulna. The method of estimating the position and size of the wedge (Fig. 233) is as follows:

A tracing is made of the radiograph of the affected limb. Normally joint surfaces are parallel—draw lines through the elbow (*ai*) and carpus (*bi*), then at the point of greatest deformity of the radius draw line (*aii*) parallel with (*ai*) and (*bii*) parallel with (*bi*). The shaded area indicates the size of the osteotomy.

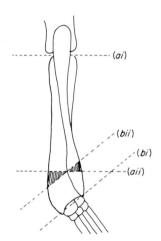

Fig. 233

The ulna must also be sectioned to allow reduction of the radius after removal of the wedge. The radial osteotomy site is stabilized with a plate. The procedure not only straightens the leg but tends to relieve concurrent elbow subluxation (Fig. 227).

PREMATURE CLOSURE OF THE DISTAL RADIAL EPIPHYSEAL PLATE (Clayton Jones & Vaughan 1970) Premature closure of the distal radial epiphyseal plate is fairly uncommon and results in shortening of the radius and forearm with an increase in the humeral-radial joint space, with consequent instability of the joint (Fig. 234a). Subluxation of the radiocarpal joint with lateral deviation of the

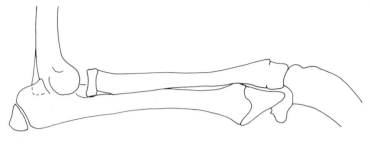

Fig. 234a

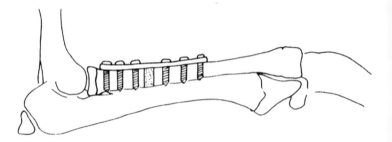

Fig. 234b

foot may also occur. The condition can be successfully treated by stabilizing the elbow joint. After transverse osteotomy of the radius 1–3 cm from its proximal end, the head of the bone is freed from its ulnar attachment and moved proximally so that it articulates snuggly again with the humeral condyles. The resultant gap at the osteotomy site is filled with a bone graft and the radius immobilized with a plate (Fig. 234b).

The operation should be delayed until the dog is 9 months of age. The alternative to lengthening the radius is to shorten the ulna. Although this causes a slight increase in limb shortening, it is technically much easier to do than the radial lengthening procedure. The caudal aspect of the ulna shaft is exposed (See Fig. 220). A section of the ulna (equal to the gap between the head of the radius and the humeral condyles) is removed (Fig. 235a). The interrosseous ligament between proximal radius and ulna is sectioned. The ulna osteotomy site is closed and stabilized with an intramedullary pin plus tension band wire (Fig. 235b).

178

Premature closure of both the radial and ulnar distal epiphyseal plates results in shortening of the radius and ulna with lateral deviation of both diaphyses. There is a tendency for the carpus to subluxate medially and produce lateral deviation of the foot. The deformity may be corrected by wedge osteotomy of the radius. The subluxation of the carpus may require reduction and immobilization in a plaster cast.

Fractures of the radius and ulna

The radius and ulna are long, straight, relatively exposed bones with little soft tissue cover, consequently, they are more vulnerable to trauma than any other in the forelimb. The majority of fractures, as might be expected, involve the distal radius and ulna and tend to be transverse in nature. However all types of fracture may be encountered and can

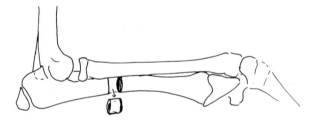

Fig. 235a

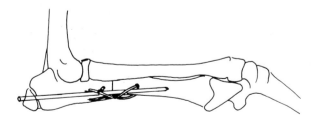

Fig. 235b

involve any part of the radius and ulna. It is convenient to classify these fractures into 3 groups, proximal, shaft, and distal fractures.

Possible sites of fracture of the proximal radius and ulna include the olecranon, the head of the radius, and the proximal ulna associated with anterior dislocation of the radial head (Monteggia fracture). These conditions are described on p. 170.

The majority of fractures involve the distal third of the radius and ulna. Shaft fractures can be treated by closed reduction and external fixation using a cast (plaster of Paris is still very popular but lighter stronger materials such as Baycast (Bayer U.K. Ltd) and Vetcast (3M) may be preferred. External fixation is indicated for greenstick fractures, undisplaced fractures and following reduction of displaced transverse fractures provided at least 50% of the fracture surfaces can be brought into contact. The cast should extend from the foot to above the elbow. The pads are left exposed so that they can be checked for warmth and swelling. In young rapidly growing puppies, the cast will need to be changed at 10–14 day intervals while in mature dogs, changes are made every 3–4 weeks once the initial swelling associated with the fracture has subsided.

Although fractures of the distal third of the radius in immature dogs heal rapidly in a cast, a serious potential complication of such fractures is premature closure of the distal ulna growth plate. Owners should be warned of this possibility and it is always worth taking a radiograph at 3 weeks to check the state of the growth plate. If closure occurs, then a section of the ulna must be removed to allow growth of the radius to continue unimpeded otherwise bowing of the radius and carpal valgus will occur. Although these deformities can be corrected by stapling or corrective osteotomy, they should be prevented from happening.

Poor reduction and/or insufficient immobilization of shaft fractures in casts may lead to malunion, or non–

union—82% of dogs referred to this clinic for treatment of non–union fractures had had their fractures plastered initially. It is generally accepted that plate fixation gives consistently good results in the treatment of fractures of the radius and ulna. The method is recommended particularly for mature dogs with overriding transverse fractures, oblique or comminuted fractures. The plate is applied to the anterior surface of the radius (Fig. 239). Generally, the distal shaft of the ulna requires no fixation because the radius is the main weight bearing bone in the forearm and tends to act as a splint for the ulna because of the interosseus attachments between the two bones.

Delayed union and non–union are common complications of fractures of the radius and ulna in Toy Poodles and other miniature breeds of dog. The non–union that develops is characterized by bone lysis and lack of callus and is termed an atrophic type of non–union. Contributary factors are:

1   The small size of these dogs which makes satisfactory immobilization of the fracture difficult, no matter whether external or internal fixation is used.

2   The potential for iatrogenic damage to bone and soft tissues which is much greater in dogs of this size.

Mini–ASIF compression plates used with cortex screws (1.5 mm or 2 mm in diameter) give good results in the treatment of both fresh and non–union fractures in toy and miniature breeds. If non–union is present, fibrous and cartilaginous callus between the fragments is excised, the fracture surfaces are freshened up and a cancellous bone graft is taken from the proximal humerus and packed into the fracture site to stimulate osteogenesis. Fixation is achieved with a mini–plate.

In some miniature dogs the diameter of the radius and ulna is too small to permit the use of a mini–plate and screws and under these circumstances an intramedullary Kirschner wire can be used for the fixation (Figs 240a, 240b, 241).

INSERTION OF AN INTRAMEDULLARY KIRSCHNER WIRE TO STABILIZE A FRACTURE OF THE RADIUS AND ULNA

This method is illustrated in Figs. 240 and 241. The fracture

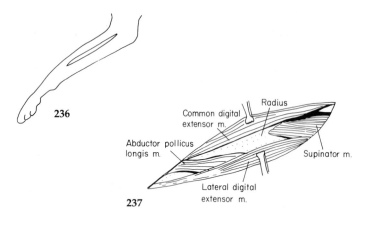

236

Radius

Common digital
extensor m.

Abductor pollicus
longis m.

Supinator m.

Lateral digital
extensor m.

237

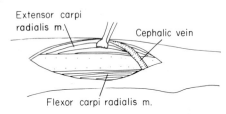

Extensor carpi
radialis m.

Cephalic vein

Flexor carpi radialis m.

238

is exposed and the medullary cavity in the proximal fragment is reamed out to a depth of about 1 cm using the tip of the Kirschner wire (Fig. 240a). The wire is then driven down through the distal fragment, keeping the carpus flexed so that the wire emerges over the dorsal aspect of the radial carpal bone (Fig. 240b). The chuck is attached to the protruding end of wire which is withdrawn sufficiently to allow fracture reduction to be completed. The Kirschner wire is then directed into the reamed medullary cavity of the proximal radius (Fig. 241).

The wire is left protruding a little (for easy retrieval after fracture healing is complete) and, it is bent back to form a hook (Fig. 241) so that the dog's ability to extend the carpus is not completely inhibited. Excess wire is cut off. After intermedullary fixation of the fracture, a plaster cast should be applied for 4 weeks to prevent any rotation at the fracture site.

The common complications of shaft fractures of the radius and ulna have already been mentioned. These are:

182

premature closure of the distal ulnar growth plate and delayed union and non–union. The fourth complication is mal union which results from failure to adequately reduce and/or immobilize the fracture during the healing process. Mal union resulting in angular deformity is corrected by wedge osteotomy. The method of estimating the position and size of the wedge is illustrated in Fig. 233.

EXPOSURE OF SHAFT FRACTURES OF THE RADIUS AND ULNA

The dog is positioned in dorsal recumbency with the fractured foreleg pulled caudally by an assistant. In this position it is easy to manipulate the leg during reduction. Both sides of the leg are accessible and it is a comfortable position for the surgeon to work in, particularly if a plate is to be inserted.

If the fracture involves the distal third of the radius, a skin incision is made over the anteromedial aspect of the radius from mid–shaft to carpus. Care is taken to avoid the cephalic vein (Fig. 238).

The extensor carpi radialis muscle is retracted laterally to expose the anterior aspect of the radius.

Fractures involving the proximal two–thirds of the radius and ulna are exposed through a skin incision made over the anteromedial aspect of the radius from the elbow to just above the carpus (Fig. 236). The deep antebrachial fascia is incised between the extensor carpi radialis muscle and flexor carpi radialis muscle to expose the radial shaft (Fig. 237). Proximally, the bone is covered by the supinator

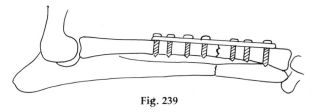

Fig. 239

muscle, this is elevated to complete exposure. The radial nerve lies deep to the supinator muscle and must be protected. Distally, the shaft of the radius is covered by the

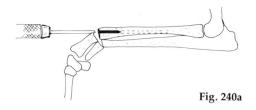

Fig. 240a

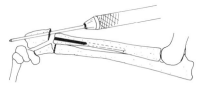

Fig. 240b

Free end of 1/M pin bent over to form hook

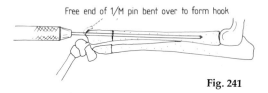

Fig. 241

abductor pollicis longus muscle which can be incised to allow application of the plate. The muscle is subsequently repaired with mattress sutures.

DISTAL RADIAL FRACTURES

Fracture separation of the distal radial epiphysis
The injury is seen in immature dogs and the distal radial epiphysis is displaced laterally causing carpal valgus (lateral deviation of the carpus (Fig. 242)). Early closed reduction should be carried out and external support provided with a plaster cast for 3 weeks while healing occurs. If treatment is delayed for more than 48 hours then reduction by closed means may prove impossible. Open reduction is carried out using a medial approach and the epiphysis stabilized with 2 K–wires in dogs under 6 months of age (Fig. 243a). The wires are removed after 4 weeks.

The distal radial growth plate normally contributes approximately 70% of the final length of the radius. Premature closure of the distal growth plate may result in

184

serious shortening of the forearm and an increase in the radio–humeral joint space with consequent elbow instability. The management of this complication is described on p. 178. In dogs over 7 months of age with little growth potential left, a wire tension band can stabilize the epiphysis (Fig. 243b). External support with a splint or cast is provided for 2–3 weeks following surgery.

Malunion of the distal radial epiphysis is occasionally encountered and this requires wedge osteotomy to correct the resultant carpal valgus deformity. The osteotomy is performed close to the growth plate and, as with more recent separations, a wire tension band and cast are used to stabilize the osteotomy.

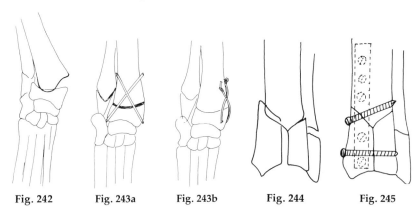

| Fig. 242 | Fig. 243a | Fig. 243b | Fig. 244 | Fig. 245 |

FRACTURES INVOLVING THE DISTAL ARTICULAR
SURFACE OF THE RADIUS AND ULNA

These are uncommon and are usually seen in dogs that have fallen from a great height. The injury is often bilateral. General principles of dealing with intra–articular fractures apply, open reduction being carried out to allow accurate reduction of the fragments. These are stabilized with lag screws or Kirschner wires and then the area is further supported with a neutralization plate or cast (Figs 244, 245).

THE CARPUS

The carpus is a composite joint (Fig. 246) supported by multiple intercarpal ligaments.

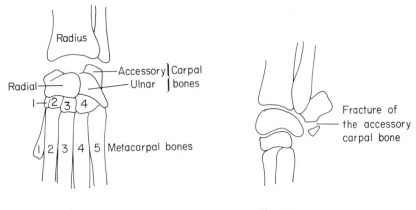

Fig. 246

Fig. 247

Fractures of the carpal bones rarely occur with the exception of the *accessory carpal bone.* A chip fracture of the ventral border of the accessory carpal bone is a common injury in the racing Greyhound which is frequently overlooked (Hickman 1975). The right leg is usually involved and the injury occurs when the dog is rounding a bend and suddenly changes direction (Bateman 1960). The injury may be dismissed initially as a sprain of the carpus and treated conservatively. However, intermittent lameness persists especially after severe exercise and there is pain on flexion of the carpus. A lateral radiograph will confirm the diagnosis (Fig. 247).

The fracture does not heal if treated conservatively because the fragment is distracted by the abductor digiti quinti muscle. In both recent and chronic cases the preferred method of treatment is surgical excision of the detached piece of bone.

Fracture of the radial carpal bone

This is a rare injury. There tends to be little displacement of the fragments and initial treatment consists of immobilization of the carpus in a plaster cast. If delayed union or non–union occurs, it is sometimes possible to compress the fragments with a small lag screw.

Fracture of the ulnar carpal bone

This fracture is occasionally seen as a complication of lateral dislocation of the radial carpal bone (see Fig. 250). Open reduction is performed and the fracture dislocation stabilized with a Kirschner wire or lag screw placed transversely through the radial and ulnar carpal bones.

Chip fractures of individual carpal bones are perhaps seen more frequently and generally the fragments should be removed to prevent carpitis developing.

EXPOSURE OF THE CARPUS

A prerequisite for accurate surgery of the extremities is a bloodless field and this is best achieved by expressing the blood from the limb with a rubber bandage followed by application of a tourniquet at, or just below, the elbow. A midline skin incision is made over the anterior aspect of the carpus. The deep antebrachial fascia is incised in the midline between the tendons of the extensor carpi radialis and common digital extensor. These tendons are retracted to allow exposure and incision of the joint capsule over the carpal bones. The synovial membrane adheres to the dorsal surfaces of individual carpal bones and must be dissected off the bones as necessary to achieve the required exposure. Following wound closure, a pressure bandage is applied before release of the tourniquet.

EXPOSURE OF THE ACCESSORY CARPAL BONE

A bloodless field is achieved as described. An oblique skin incision is made over the lateral surface of the carpus, extending over the radial carpal bone to the proximal end of the 5th metacarpal bone. Fascia along the cranial border of the adductor digiti quinti muscle is incised together with the palmar carpal transverse ligament. The abductor muscle is retracted to expose the accessory carpal bone.

Dislocation and sub-luxation of the radiocarpal joint

Dislocations or sub-luxations of the radiocarpal joint are usually caused by a fall. The radius is displaced cranial to the radial carpal bone and there is often damage to the medial collateral ligament which causes lateral deviation of the foot (Fig. 248a).

After closed reduction, joint stability may be restored by immobilizing the carpus in a plaster cast for at least 4 weeks. If instability persists and there is deviation of the foot, then surgical replacement of the medial collateral ligament is carried out using a wire prosthesis (Fig. 248b). Occasionally carpal arthrodesis is indicated, (Fig. 252), when there has been extensive damage to the collateral ligaments.

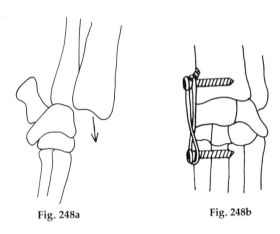

Fig. 248a   Fig. 248b

Rupture of the plantar ligament of the carpus

Rupture of the plantar ligament of the carpus (Fig. 249a) is usually caused by a fall. The carpus 'drops' when the dog takes weight on the affected leg and the joint can be hyper-extended on palpation. Carpal posture may improve following external support in a plaster cast but this is usually transient. The plantar ligaments can be replaced with a wire tension band (18 or 20 gauge wire) fixed in tunnels drilled through the accessory carpal bone and through the head of the 5th metacarpal bone (Fig. 249b). External support with a cast or splint should be provided for 4 weeks following surgery. If the procedure fails then partial carpal arthrodesis can always be carried out using intra-medullary pins (Slocum & Devine 1982 (Fig. 249c)) or a 'T' plate (Brinker *et al* 1983 (Fig. 249d)). These procedures are

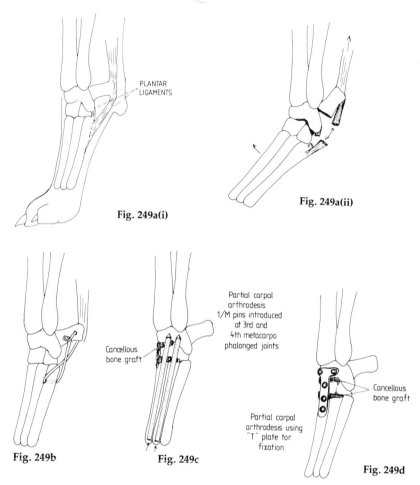

PLANTAR
LIGAMENTS

Fig. 249a(i)

Fig. 249a(ii)

Fig. 249b

Cancellous
bone graft

Fig. 249c

Partial carpal
arthrodesis
1/M pins introduced
at 3rd and
4th metacarpo
phalonged joints

Partial carpal
arthrodesis using
"T" plate for
fixation

Cancellous
bone graft

Fig. 249d

used only if a stressed lateral radiograph of the carpus
reveals hyperextension at the intercarpal or carpo-meta-
carpal joints.

Dislocation of the radial carpal bone (Fig. 250)

Dislocation of the radial carpal bone is an uncommon
injury. Open reduction is usually necessary as the bone
tends to rotate on its horizontal axis. Normally a stable
reduction is achieved. However, if it is difficult to maintain
the bone in position, a small pin can be used for fixation
(Fig. 251). After reduction the carpus is immobilized in a
plaster cast for 4 weeks.

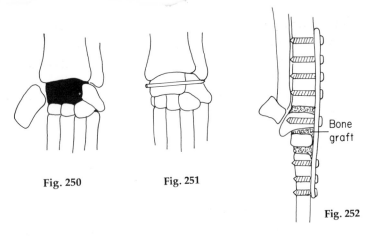

Fig. 250   Fig. 251

Bone
graft

Fig. 252

Carpal arthrodesis

The main indications for carpal arthrodesis are the relief of pain associated with osteoarthritis and the restoration of stability following dislocation of the joint.

TECHNIQUE
A bloodless field is achieved by expressing the blood from the limb with a rubber bandage followed by the application of a tourniquet above the elbow. A skin incision is made over the medial aspect of the carpus. The incision extends from the distal third of the radius to the distal third of the metacarpus. The joint capsule is incised and reflected laterally with the digital extensor tendons. The articular cartilage is removed and the joint spaces packed with cancellous bone taken from the proximal humerus. A plate is applied to the anterior aspect of the joint (Fig. 252). For optimal stability, 3 screws should be placed in the 3rd metacarpal bone, one in the radial carpal bone and four in the distal radius (Fig. 252) External support with a plaster cast should be given for at least one month.

Dogs manage well following carpal arthrodesis and should resume a 'normal' action.

Fractures of the metacarpal bones

Fractures of the metacarpal bones are common in dogs and are usually caused when the foot is crushed by a car wheel.

190

Consequently the fractures may be multiple, comminuted or compound. However, the prognosis is invariably good and the fractures heal well following closed reduction and immobilization in a plaster cast. Intramedullary pinning (Whittick 1974) is occasionally used in grossly displaced fractures (Fig. 249c).

Fractures of the phalanges

Fractures of the phalanges occur in the racing Greyhound due to a rapid or inco-ordinate turn placing torsional stress on the phalanx but in other breeds the fracture is more commonly caused by a crush injury. Closed reduction and external support in a plaster cast is a satisfactory form of treatment for all dogs except the racing Greyhound. If the Greyhound is to regain its form best results are obtained by treating the fracture by open reduction and fixation with a lag screw or wire sutures. If lameness persists after the fracture has healed performance may improve after amputation of the distal phalanx to relieve pressure on the fracture site.

Dislocation of the interphalangeal joints 'knocked-up toe'
(Davies 1958; Bateman 1960; Hickman 1975)

Dislocation of the interphalangeal joints is an injury which is frequently encountered in the racing Greyhound. The digits of the left forefoot, particularly the fifth, are usually affected.

Dislocation and subluxations of the interphalangeal joints seldom remain stable following reduction in the Greyhound. Although attention has been directed to affecting stabilization by internal fixation the results are disappointing and consequently the trend in to relieve pressure on the joint.

Treatment of a dislocation or subluxation of the distal interphalangeal joint comprises reduction followed by removal of the nail. The dog is given four weeks' rest before training is resumed. If lameness persists then amputation is performed through the distal end of the second phalanx and the third phalanx is removed. Care is taken to conserve the pad.

191

Dislocations and subluxation of the proximal inter-phalangeal joint are best treated by arthrodesis of the joint in the normal standing position. Arthrodesis is performed by removal of the articular cartilage and fixation achieved with wire suture. The nail is also removed to relieve stress on the joint. If lameness persists complete amputation of the third phalanx is carried out.

Fractures of the proximal volar sesamoid (Davies, Bellinger & Turner 1969)

These fractures are seen mainly in the racing Greyhound and the 2nd and 7th sesamoid on the right fore are most frequently fractured. The fracture tends to be transverse but can be comminuted. It may heal if the foot is immobilized in a cast with the digits in flexion but fibrous non–unions often persist and Bateman (1959) recommends surgical excision of the fractured sesamoid to prevent lameness.

Section of the digital flexor tendons

The injury is most frequently caused by the dog stepping on broken glass. The wound occurs between the digital pads on the caudal aspect of the metacarpus or metatarsus. There is profuse haemorrhage and the natural tendency is to control this with sutures and bandage and the important tendon injury is missed. Section of the superficial digital flexor tendon is of little significance but if the deep digital flexor is cut, then flattening of one or more digits occurs. The severed tendon should be repaired (see page 265) and post-operatively a bandage is applied for 3–4 weeks to maintain the foot in a semi-flexed position to ease tension on the sutures.

Amputation of the forelimb

The indications for amputation of the forelimb include:
1 Gross trauma.
2 Gangrene.
3 Paralysis.
4 Osteomyelitis.

5 Neoplasia.

Although complete amputation of the forelimb including the scapula can be performed (Harvey 1974) it is simpler to amputate the limb through the proximal third of the humerus (Hickman 1964).

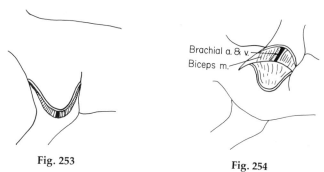

Fig. 253

Fig. 254

A semicircular skin incision is made on the lateral aspect of the limb (Fig. 253). The limb is then lifted by an assistant and a similar incision is made on the medial side of the limb. The skin flap is reflected and the brachial artery and vein identified between the triceps and the biceps muscle (Fig. 254). Both vessels are ligated and severed. (Early ligation of these vessels reduces the amount of haemorrhage during the operation.)

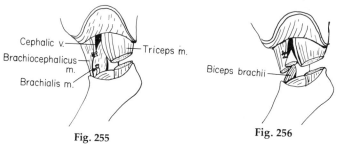

Fig. 255

Fig. 256

The limb is lowered, the lateral skin flap is elevated and the cephalic vein ligated (Fig. 255). The common tendon of insertion of the triceps is severed and the muscle mass reflected proximally to expose the brachialis and radial nerve (Fig. 255). The nerve and brachialis muscle are severed to complete exposure of the distal humerus (Fig. 256).

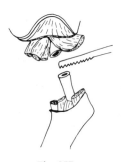

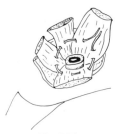

Fig. 257a   Fig. 257b

The muscles are then bluntly pushed back from the shaft with a swab until the proximal third is exposed. Amputation is completed by sawing through the humerus at this level (Fig. 257a).

Dead space between the muscle bellies is closed with a series of purse string sutures started close to the cut end of the bone and working towards the severed ends of the muscles (Fig. 257b). Finally the ends of the muscles are sutured together with horizontal mattress sutures and the skin flaps closed in the same manner.

REFERENCES

Ball D.C. (1968) A case of medial luxation of the canine shoulder joint and its surgical correction. *Vet. Rec.* **83**, 195.

Bateman J.K. (1960) *Vet. Rec.* **72**, 895.

Bateman J.K. (1959) Fracture of the Sesamoid Bones in the Dog. *Vet.Rec.* **71**, 101.

Bennet D. & Vaughan L.C. (1976) The use of muscle relocation techniques in the treatment of peripheral nerve injuries in dogs and cats *J. small Anim. Pract.* **17**, 99.

Birkhead R. (1967) Osteochondritis dissecans in the humeral head of the dog. *Nord. Vet. Med.* **19**, 294.

Boyd H.B. & Boals J.C. (1969) The Monteggia lesion. *Clinical Orthopaedics and Related Research,* **66**, 94.

Braden T.D. (1975) Surgical correction of humeral fractures In: *Current Techniques in Small Animal Surgery.* Ed. Bojrab, M.J., Lea & Febiger, Philadelphia.

Brinker W.O. (1974) Fractures of the Humerus In: *Canine Surgery,* 2nd Archibald ed. p. 1019. American Vet Publications Inc. Drawer KK, Santa Barbara, California.

Brinker W.O., Piermattei P.L. & Flo G. L. (1983) *Handbook of Small Animal Orthopaedics and Fracture Treatment.* W.B. Saunders Company, Philadelphia.

Campbell J.R. (1968) Shoulder lameness in the dog. *J. small Anim. Pract.* **9,** 189.

Caywood D., Wallace L.J., Johnston G.R. (1977) The use of a Plastic Plate for repair of a comminuted scapular body fracture in a dog. *J. Am. Anim. Hosp.Ass.,* **13,** 176.

Cheli R. (1976) Surgical treatment of fractures of the scapula in the dog and cat. *Folia vet. lat.* **6,** 189.

Clayton-Jones D.G. & Vaughan L.C. (1972) Disturbances in the growth of the radius in dogs. *J. small Anim. Pract.,* **11,** 453.

Corley E.A. (1968) Genetic aspects of canine elbow dysplasia. *J. Am. Vet. Med. Ass.* **153,** 543.

Craig P.H. & Riser W.H. (1965) Osteochondritis dissecans in the proximal humerus of the dog. *J. Am. Vet. Rad. Soc.,* **6,** 40.

David P.E., Bellenger C.R. and Turner D.M. (1969) Fractures of the Sesamoid Bones in the Greyhound. *Aust. Vet. J.* **45,** 15.

Davies J.J. (1958) *Vet. Rec.* **70,** 660.

De Angelis M. & Schwartz A. (1970) Surgical correction of cranial dislocation of the scapulohumeral joint in a dog. *J. Am. Vet. Med. Ass.* **156,** 435.

Denny H.R. (1976) The treatment of growth disturbances of the canine radius and ulna. *The Veterinary Annual,* 16th edn, p. 170. Wright Scientechnic, Bristol.

Denny H.R. & Gibbs C. (1980) The surgical treatment of osteochondritis dissecans and ununited coronoid process in the canine elbow. *J. small Anim. Pract.* **21,** 323.

Denny H.R. (1983) Condylar Fractures of the Humerus in the dog: a review of 133 cases. *J. small Anim. Pract.* **24,** 185.

Evans P.J. (1968) Shoulder dysplasia in a labrador. *J. small Anim. Pract.* **9,** 189.

Fackelman G.E. (1972) The current status of ASIF technique in large animals. *Proc. 18th A. Conv. Am. Ass. Equine Pract.,* p. 325.

Griffiths R.C. (1968) Osteochondritis dissecans of the canine shoulder. *J. Am. Vet. Med. Ass.* **153,** 1733.

Grøndelen J. & Rørvik A.M. (1980) Arthrosis in the elbow joint of young rapidly growing dogs IV. Ununited ancroneal process. A follow up investigation of operated dogs. *Nord. Vet. Med.* **32,** 212.

Hanlon G.F. (1969) Additional radiographic observations on elbow dysplasia in the dog. *J. Am. Vet. Med. Ass.* **155,** 2045.

Harvey C.E. (1974) Complete forequarter amputation in the dog and cat. *J. Am. Anim. Hosp. Ass.* **10,** 125.

Hickman J. (1964) *Veterinary Orthopaedics.* Oliver & Boyd, Edinburgh and London.

Hickman J. (1975) *J. small Anim. Pract. Greyhound injuries.* **16,** 455.

Hohn R.B. *et al.* (1971) Surgical stabilization of recurrent luxations. *Vet. Clinics of North America.* **1:3,** 537.

Holt P.E. (1978) Longitudinal fracture of the scapula in a dog *Vet. Rec.* **102,** 311.

Hufford T.J., Olmstead M.L. & Butler H.C. (1975) Contracture of the infraspinatus muscle and surgical correction in 2 dogs. *J. Am. Anim. Hosp. Ass.* **11,** 613.

Jones D.G.C. & Vaughan L.C. (1970) The surgical treatment of osteochondritis dissecans of the humeral head in dogs. *J. small Anim. Pract.* **11**, 803.

Knight G.S. (1956) The use of transfixion screws for internal fixation of fractures in small animals *Vet Rec.* **68**, 415.

Knight G.S. (1959) Internal fixation of the fractured lateral humeral condyle *Vet. Rec.* **71**, 667.

Leighton R.L. (1969) Open reduction of the canine shoulder joint. *J. Am. Vet. Med. Ass.* **155**, 1987.

Leighton R.L. (1978) Osteochondritis dissecans of the elbow in a dog. *Vet. Med. Small Anim. Clin.* **73**, 311.

Ljunggren G., Cawley A.J. & Archibald J. (1966) The elbow dysplasias in the dog. *J. Am. Vet. Med. Ass.* **148**, 887.

McCurnin D.M., Slusher R. & Grier R.L. (1976) A medical approach to the canine elbow joint. *J. Am. Anim. Hosp. Ass.* **12**, 475.

Neal T.M. (1975) Fractures of the Radius and Ulna in Current Techniques in Small Animal Surgery. Ed. Bojrab, M.J. Lea 7 Febiger, Philadelphia.

Newton C.D. (1974) Surgical management of distal ulnar physeal growth disturbances in dogs. *J. Am. Vet. Med. Ass.* **164**, 479.

O'Brien T.R., Morgan J.P. & Suter P.F. (1971) Epiphyseal plate injury in the dog: a radiographic study of growth disturbance in the forelimb. *J. Small Anim. Pract.* **12**, 19.

Olsson S.E. (1975) Lameness in the dog. *Proceedings Am. Anim. Hosp. Ass.* **42**, 363.

Parkes L.J., Riser W.H. & Martin C.L. (1966) Clinicopathologic conference. *J. Anim. Vet. Ass.* **149**, 1086.

Payne–Johnson M. & Lewis D.G. (1981) A technique for fixation of intercondylar humeral fractures in immature small dogs *J. small Anim. Pract.* **22**, 293.

Piermattei D.C. & Greeley R.G. (1979) *An Atlas of Surgical Approaches to the Bones of the Dog and Cat.* 2nd Edn. W.B. Saunders Company, Philadelphia, London, Toronto.

Shuttleworth A.C. (1938) *Vet. Jnl.* **94**, 275.

Slocum B. & Devine T. (1982) Practical carpal fusion in the dog. *J. Am. Vet. Med. Ass.* **180**, 1204.

Smith C.W., Stowater J.L. (1975) Osteochondritis dissecans of the canine shoulder joint. A review of 35 cases. *J. Am. Anim. Hosp. Ass.* **11**, 658.

Vaughan L.C. (1967) Dislocation of the shoulder joint in the dog and cat. *J. small Anim. Pract.* **8**, 45.

Vaughan L.C. (1976) Growth plate defects in dogs. *Vet. Rec.* **98**, 185.

Vaughan L.C. & Jones D.G.C. (1968) Osteochondritis dissecans of the head of the humerus in dogs. *J. small Anim. Pract.* **9**, 283.

Vaughan L.C. & Jones D.G.C. (1969) Congenital dislocation of the shoulder joint in the dog. *J. small Anim. Pract.* **10**, 1.

Vaughan L.C. (1979) Muscle and tendon injuries in dogs *J. small Anim. Pract.* **20**, 711–736.

Walker R.G. & Hickman J. (1958) Injuries of the elbow in the dog, *Vet. Rec.* **70**, 1191.

Whittick W.G. (1974) *Canine Orthopaedics.* Lea & Febiger, Philadelphia.

Wood A.K.W., Bath M.C. & Mason T.A. (1975) Osteochondritis dissecans of the distal humerus in a dog. *Vet. Rec.* **91**, 489.

Chapter 5
The Hindlimb

Examination of the dog with hindleg lameness

A protocol for examination of the lame dog has already been given at the beginning of Chapter 4. Common or well recognized causes of hindleg lameness are listed below. These should be kept in mind when the examination is carried out.

TRAUMATIC CONDITIONS OF THE HINDLEG

Pelvis
Fracture.

Hip
Acetabular fractures.
Fractures of the femoral head or neck±trochanteric fractures.
Hip disloction.

Femur
Fractures of the proximal femur—see above.
Fractures of the shaft.
Supracondylar and condylar fractures.

Stifle
Rupture of
   (a) anterior cruciate ligament ± damage to medial meniscus.
   (b) collateral ligament.
   (c) straight patellar ligament.
Traumatic dislocations of the patella.
Traumatic dislocations of the stifle.
Avulsion of the tendon of origin of the long digital extensor muscle.
Fractures of the distal femur—see above.

Fractures of the patella.
Fractures of the proximal tibia
  avulsion of the tibial crest.
  separation of the proximal epiphysis of the tibia.

Tibia
Fractures of the proximal tibia—see above.
Fractures of the shaft.
Distal tibial fractures
  malleolar fractures.
  separation of distal epiphysis

Hock
Malleolar fracture.
Rupture of collateral ligaments } dislocation of the
Severe abrasion injury. tibiotarsal joint.
Fractures of the os calcis.
Injuries of the Achilles tendon.
Intertarsal subluxation (rupture of plantar ligaments
  (Shelties, Collies).
Fracture of the central tarsal bone.
Fractures of the metatarsus and digits.

DEVELOPMENTAL DISORDERS CAUSING HIND LEG
LAMENESS

Hip

Hip dysplasia	Most large breeds, Alsatians, Labradors, Retrievers especially
Legge Perthes Disease	Terriers

Stifle

Congenital medial luxation of the patella	Small breeds, C.K.C. Spaniels currently seen most frequently.
Osteochondritis dissecans	Wolfhounds, Labradors, Retrievers, Alsatians, Greyhounds.
Genu valgum	Giant breeds

198

Hock

Osteochondritis dissecans	Labradors, Retrievers, Rottweilers, Wolfhounds

1 Lumbosacral lesions—'cauda equina syndrome'.
2 Osteoarthritis of hip.
3 Osteosarcoma distal femur.
4 Osteoarthritis of stifle.
5 Bilateral anterior cruciate ligament rupture in overweight dogs.
6 Osteosarcoma proximal tibia.

PHYSICAL EXAMINATION FOR HINDLEG LAMENESS

The owner or an assistant should steady the dog's head while examination of the hind quarters is being carried out. The stages in the examination given here relate to specific injuries or conditions and obviously do not have to be carried to these lengths in every case, however, each joint should be palpated systematically and both legs carefully compared. Do not omit the rest of the examination when the diagnosis appears obvious. For example, a young Labrador may have hip dysplasia but it is quite possible for that animal to have osteochondritis dissecans in its hock joints as well.

The palpable areas of the pelvis and hip are illustrated in Fig. 258a, the external landmarks include the iliac crests, the

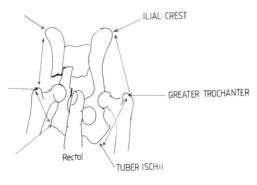

Fig. 258a

199

greater trochanter and the tuber ischii. On rectal examination, the ischium, medial acetabulum and pelvis can be
palpated. When traumatic injuries of the pelvis and hip are
suspected, i.e. pelvic fractures, dislocation of the hip,
fractures of the femoral head and neck, then feel the
external palpable landmarks of the pelvis. Compare their
relationship with the greater trochanter, (Fig. 258a) and
check for differences between each side of the pelvis. Rectal
examination can also be useful to confirm pelvic fractures.
These fractures are occasionally complicated by bladder
rupture or injury to the urinary tract. If there is any doubt
about the integrity of the bladder or urethra then cysto-
graphy and/or urethrography should be undertaken as
necessary.

Compare the length of both hind legs by gripping them
just proximal to the stifles, then extend them. Most hip
dislocations result in craniodorsal displacement of the
femoral head in relation to the acetabulum so the affected
leg will be shorter.

Remember that the dog with a fracture of the femoral
neck will also have apparent shortening of the affected leg
but there is more pain and crepitus evident on manipulation
than in a dislocation.

Developmental disorders of the hip

The clinical signs associated with hip dysplasia include poor
muscling of the hind quarters with laxity, pain and crepitus
on manipulation of the hips. There are specific tests for hip
laxity. Make the dog walk while your hands are held firmly
over each greater trochanter. If the hips are very loose,
crepitus will be felt as the femoral head slips in and out of
the acetabulum. Lie the dog on its side, grip the uppermost
leg proximal to the stifle with one hand and try to raise the
femoral head out of the acetabulum while keeping the
leg parallel to the ground. At the same time place the other
hand firmly over the greater trochanter and try and bounce
the femoral head in and out of the acetabulum. A definite
'clunking' sound will be appreciated if the hip is loose.

Try and elicit the Ortolani sign. This can be done with the

dog standing or lying on its side. Grip the stifle, adduct the leg and then push the femur towards the hip joint. If there is laxity of the joint the femoral head will ride up on the dorsal rim of the acetabulum and then click back into its normal position as pressure on the lower leg is released.

Dogs with hip dysplasia often have taut pectineus muscles. Lie the dog on its back, abduct both hind legs. It should be possible to bring the stifles almost in contact with the ground. Check the pectineus muscle during the procedure (it is the most prominent muscle over the medial side of the hip)—does it become excessively taut or painful? Although many older Alsatians presented with hindleg weakness will have radiographic evidence of hip dysplasia their clinical signs are not usually due to this but are caused by a spinal disorder, chronic degenerative radiculomyelopathy (see p. 86).

Chronic hip pain particularly on abduction of the joint in Terrier breeds under a year of age is generally due to Legge Perthes disease.

Femoral shaft fractures should be obvious on clinical examination. Supracondylar fractures of the femur are not always unstable and are sometimes missed on a cursory examination. If there is swelling and pain following trauma, take a radiograph and this should confirm the fracture if present.

The gradual development of a painful swelling involving the distal femur or proximal tibia in larger breeds is most likely to be caused by an osteosarcoma.

The stifle

The palpable areas of the stifle are the distal femur, proximal tibia, tibial crest, patella and straight patellar ligament. Compare both stifles for differences in size. In chronic anterior cruciate ligament injuries the medial side of the stifle over the proximal tibia becomes thickened. Crepitus on manipulation of the stifle is usually due to osteoarthritis. Distinct 'clicking' noises coming from the stifle are heard in dogs with anterior cruciate ligament rupture when the femoral condyles slip in and out of their normal position on the menisci. Check the stability of the stifle joint; the commonest cause of lameness is rupture of the anterior cruciate ligament and this diagnosis is confirmed by demonstration of the anterior draw movement (Fig. 258b).

The collateral ligaments of the stifle can also be damaged and give instability. If, for example, the medial collateral ligament is ruptured it is possible to displace the tibia laterally on the femur. The stifle joint can also be hinged open on the medial side (Fig. 258c).

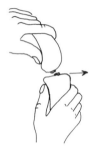

Anterior draw movement

Fig. 258b

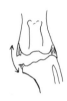

Rupture of
medial collateral
ligament

Fig. 258c

The position of the patella should be checked. Upward displacement or laxity of the straight patellar ligament is associated with injuries to the ligament or fractures of the patella.

The most common developmental disorder of the stifle is congenital medial luxation of the patella. Dogs with intermittent patella luxation walk normally until the patella luxates, the leg may then be carried in a semi–flexed position for a few paces. The dog stretches the leg and is generally able to reduce the luxation itself and consequently resumes a normal action. Permanent medial luxation gives a crouching hind leg action with lateral bowing of the stifle. Check if the patella is riding in the trochlea, can it be displaced medially; the best position to attempt displacement is with the stifle extended or slightly flexed. Compare the position of the tibial crests.

Dogs with permanent medial luxation of the patella will generally have a tibial crest which is rotated 15–90° medial to the long axis of the stifle.

Hock

Most areas of the hock can be palpated. Check the range of hock flexion; it should be possible to touch the anterior aspect of the tibia with the tips of the toes when the joint is fully flexed. A straight hock with a limited range of flexion is a feature of osteochondritis dissecans. If the hock is 'dropped' giving a plantegrade stance, check the Achilles tendon for rupture or avulsion from the os calcis. Also check the os calcis for fracture.

Dropping of the hock with caudal bowing of the intertarsal region is seen in overweight Shelties and Collies when rupture of the plantar ligaments causes an intertarsal subluxation.

Fractures of the central tarsal bone are seen in the Racing Greyhound and cause marked swelling and pain. If the clinical and radiological examination fails to reveal a cause of hind leg lameness, it is always worth checking the lumbosacral junction. Palpate this area and extend the junction by extending the hind legs (does this cause pain?). Take a lateral radiograph of the lumbosacral junction to check for the lesions of the cauda equina which can cause a hind leg lameness (see p. 114).

ORTHOPAEDIC CAUSES OF EXERCISE INTOLERANCE AND COLLAPSE

The conditions which cause exercise intolerance and collapse all impede the function of two or more limbs. Most of the conditions are described in more detail in other sections of the book. They are listed here as a guide to diagnosis.
1   One of the earliest is the Swimmer syndrome in puppies.
2   Spinal conditions:
(a) Congenital defects, e.g. Hemivertebrae—screw tail

breeds, Bulldogs, etc. Hindleg ataxia+collapse at 3–4 months.

(b) Cervical spondylopathy (Wobbler Syndrome)—Great Danes (4 months onwards). Dobermans (1–12 years).

(c) Spinal haemorrhage.
(d) Infarction due to fibrocartilaginous emboli. Young dogs.

(e) Spinal trauma.

(f) Atlanto–axial subluxation—Yorkshire Terriers, Poms. under 1 year.

(g) Discs—Dachshunds especially.

(h) Cauda equina lesions—older dogs, larger breeds.

(i) Chronic Degenerative Radiculomyelopathy—CDRM (older Alsations especially).

Peripheral neuropathies
Giant Axonal Neuropathy—young Alsatians.
Distal Denervating Disease—young dogs, larger breeds.
Progressive Axonopathy—Boxers.

3   *Nutritional bone diseases*
Juvenile osteoporosis (Nutritional Secondary Hyperparathyroidism).
Pups 3–4 months of age, pain, lameness, reluctance to move.

Skeletal scurvy (hypertrophic osteodystrophy)
Large and giant breeds—4–6 months.
Metaphyses of long bones enlarged and painful. Intermittent pyrexia.

4   Developmental disorders—
Hip dysplasia
Legge perthes
Patella luxation
Osteochondritis dissecans

5   Degenerative joint disease—
Secondary to developmental joint disorders.
Secondary to joint injury, e.g. bilateral anterior cruciate ligament rupture.
Polyarthritis, e.g. Rheumatoid.

6   Bilateral fractures, e.g. Avulsion of tibial crests.
Bilateral ligamentous injury, e.g. Avulsion of straight patellar ligament.

204

Avulsion of gastrocnemeus tendons.
Rupture of plantar ligaments of hocks.
7 Myopathies.

Pelvic fractures

The majority of pelvic fractures in the dog will heal satis-
factorily with conservative treatment (Grondalen 1969).
However, in some cases malalignment and/or instability of
the fragments may result in a prolonged recovery period,
narrowing of the pelvic canal or limited hip movement.

In recent years there has been growing interest in the
open reduction and internal fixation of pelvic fractures
(Leighton 1968; Robins et al 1973; Morris 1970; Kirkbride &
Carter 1970; Wheaton et al 1973; Whittick 1974; Brown &
Biggart 1975; Brinker 1975; Pond 1975; Hauptman et al 1976).

The open reduction of pelvic fractures is not without
hazard and it has been said 'that no other type of fracture
lends itself to iatrogenic trauma with so little to show for
surgical interference as does the fractured pelvis' (Whittick,
1974).

In 1978 the author reviewed a series of pelvic fracture
cases. The purpose of the review was to classify pelvic
fractures, compare the results of conservative and surgical
treatment and establish criteria for adopting either method
of treatment.

One hundred and twenty-three dogs had pelvic fracture
and the cause of the injury was a road traffic accident in all
cases. The majority of dogs were under 3 years of age.
Trauma is haphazard in its effects and extent and this is
reflected in the great variety in the position and number of
pelvic fracture sites recorded. There was a total of 66 com-
binations of fracture site and no fixed pattern of fracture
could be predicted.

The most common complications associated with fracture
of the pelvis were: dislocation of the hip in 11% of cases,
fracture of the femur in 8% and sciatic nerve paralysis in
2%. Only one dog had a ruptured bladder, while two had
rupture of the urethra.

The results of treatment of pelvic fractures were assessed

with reference to 40 cases which were managed conservatively and 28 surgically. The follow-up period ranged from 1 to 5 years. Of the dogs treated conservatively, 75% made complete recoveries while the other 25% were either occasionally lame or a slight limp persisted. A slightly higher percentage (78%) of dogs managed surgically made complete recoveries. The recovery period was considerably reduced in most cases. The other 22% were either occasionally lame or had a slight limp, while one dog was severely lame with a permanent sciatic nerve paralysis.

It is difficult to make accurate comparisons between the results of treatment for specific fracture sites because of the number of variable factors, particularly with regard to site and combination of other pelvic fractures. The results of conservative and surgical treatment for sacro-iliac separation or fracture were virtually identical. All the animals except one in the conservative group which had a slight limp made full recoveries in an average time of 6 weeks. Intense pain associated with the injury was rapidly alleviated by surgery.

The duration of lameness after the accident in dogs with fractures of the ilium was reduced by surgical treatment to an average of 3 weeks as compared to 8 weeks for conservative treatment. All the surgical cases made complete recoveries as did the dogs in the conservative group, except for two animals which remained slightly lame.

The recovery period for undisplaced fractures of the acetabulum was slightly reduced by surgical treatment to an average of 6 weeks as opposed to 7 weeks for conservative management. Of cases treated surgically 70% made complete recoveries compared with 55% treated conservatively.

Some dogs with multiple pelvic fractures, particularly those with marked displacement of the iliac or acetabular fragments, had prolonged recovery periods of 6–9 months when managed conservatively; this period was greatly reduced by surgical treatment to an average of 6 weeks.

In conclusion, the majority of dogs with pelvic fractures will recover with conservative treatment. However, the recovery period can be reduced by surgical treatment especially in dogs with multiple bilateral fractures, dogs with fractures of the ilium associated with fracture of the ipsilateral pubis and ischium, and in dogs with displaced fractures of the acetabulum.

CONSERVATIVE TREATMENT OF PELVIC FRACTURES

Owners are instructed to rest the dog for a period of one month. If it is unable to take weight on the hind limbs a foam rubber mattress should be provided for the animal to lie on. Massage and regular turning should be encouraged to prevent the development of decubitus ulcers. Owners are also advised to observe that the dog continues to urinate and defaecate and what measures to take to assist it to do so.

THE SURGICAL TREATMENT OF PELVIC FRACTURES

The weight bearing areas of the pelvis are the sacro–iliac joints the ilium and the acetabulum. These are the areas that may require internal fixation. The pubis and ischium are non weight bearing areas in which fractures do not require fixation as a general rule. Simultaneous reduction of pubic and ischial fractures tends to occur once fractures of weight bearing areas of the pelvis are reduced and fixed.

The criteria for surgical treatment are pelvic fractures characterized by one or more of the following:

1   Fracture of the acetabulum with displacement of the articular surfaces.

2   Fracture of the ipsilateral ilium, ischium and pubis with resultant instability of the hip joint.

3   Marked displacement of fragments into the pelvic canal.

4   Multiple bilateral fractures of weight bearing areas of the pelvis.

5   Multiple fractures of the pelvis and hind limbs.

The open reduction and internal fixation of pelvic fractures is difficult. Reduction should be undertaken as soon as the animal is considered to be in a fit state for surgery. If surgery is delayed for more than a week, reduction of the fragments may prove impossible due to muscle contraction.

Sacro–iliac Separation or Fracture

A sacro-iliac separation or fracture (Fig. 259) may be stabilized after open or closed reduction by the use of an intra-

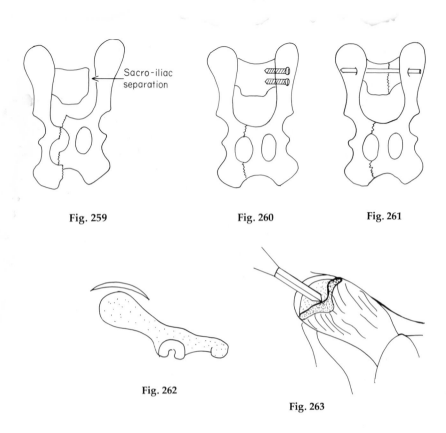

Fig. 259

Fig. 260

Fig. 261

Sacro-iliac separation

Fig. 262

Fig. 263

medullary pin driven transversely through the wing of the ilium into the contralateral ilium (Fig. 261). The pin is passed over the dorsal surface of the sacrum (Leighton 1968; Whittick 1974). Lag screws (Fig. 260) can also be used for fixation of the sacro–iliac junction and provide optimal stability (Brinker 1975; Pond 1975; Hauptman *et al* 1976).

The surgical approach to the sacro–iliac joint and wing of the ilium has been described by Piermattei & Greeley (1966). A skin incision is made directly over the crest of the ilium (Fig. 262) the cutaneous trunci muscle and gluteal fascia are incised to reveal the middle gluteal muscle and iliac crest. The wing of the ilium is exposed by elevating the origin of the middle gluteal muscle (Fig. 263). The muscles which cover the sacro–iliac joint and insert on the medial surface of the crest and wing of the ilium (Iliocostalis and longissimus groups) are usually severely damaged and little elevation is required to expose the joint.

208

The sacro–iliac joint is reduced and maintained in position with reduction forceps gripping the lateral surface of the ilium and medial dorsal aspect of the wing of the sacrum; alternatively a small Kirschner pin is temporarily driven through the wing of the ilium into the sacrum. The wing of the ilium is then lagged to the sacrum with one or, preferably, two screws. Careful reference is made to the ventro-dorsal radiograph of the pelvis to ensure that the screws chosen are of the correct length and do not penetrate the neural canal.

Lag screws are preferred for simple sacro–iliac separation, but when the separation is associated with a sagittal fracture of the sacrum (Fig. 261), the fracture is stabilized by transfixing the wings of the ilium with a pin because there is usually insufficient bone left on the medial aspect of the sacral fracture to permit the use of a screw without penetration of the neural canal.

Fractures of the ilium

A variety of methods of internal fixation have been used for the treatment of fractures of the ilium (Brinker 1965; Leighton 1968; Brown & Biggart 1975; Robins *et al* 1973; Whittick 1974 and Brinker 1975).

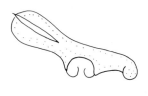

Fig. 264

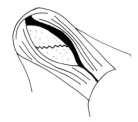

Fig. 265

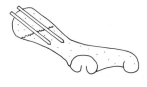

Fig. 266

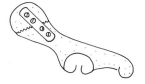

Fig. 267

Fractures of the wing of the ilium are exposed through a lateral skin incision (Fig. 264). The middle gluteal muscle is then split in the direction of its fibres to reveal the fracture (Fig. 265).

Although two pins can be used to stabilize the fracture (Brinker 1975) (Fig. 266), a plate is the preferred method of fixation (Fig. 267).

Fractures of the shaft of the ilium may be stabilized with a plate (Robins *et al* 1973; Brown & Biggart 1975) or alternatively lag screws or Kirshner pins and a wire suture may be used for the fixation of oblique fractures (Brinker 1975).

Exposure of the shaft of the ilium is illustrated in Figs 268–271.

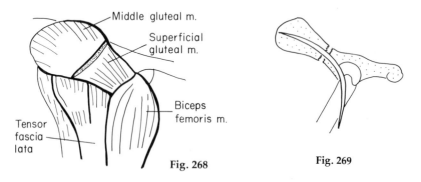

Fig. 268

Fig. 269

A lateral approach with dorsal reflection of the gluteal muscles is used to expose the ilium (Brinker 1975) (Figs 268–271). A skin incision is made from the iliac crest and extended caudally over the greater trochanter (Fig. 269).

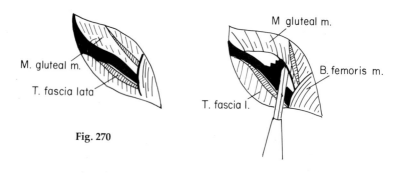

Fig. 270

Fig. 271

The incision is continued through the subcutaneous fat and gluteal fascia to expose the aponeurosis between the middle gluteal muscle and the tensor fascia lata (Fig. 270). The two muscles are separated and the lateral surface of the body and wing of the ilium exposed by dorsal reflection of the middle and deep gluteal muscles (Fig. 271). The application of bone holding forceps should be done with care to avoid crushing the sciatic nerve which runs close to the medial aspect of the ilium.

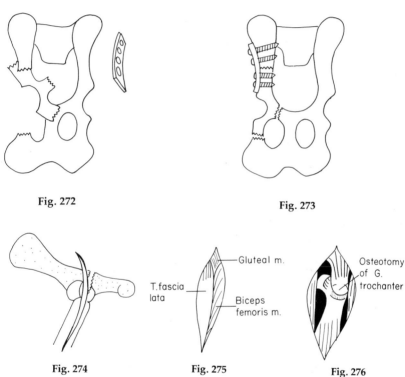

Fig. 272

Fig. 273

Fig. 274

Fig. 275

T.fascia lata

Gluteal m.

Biceps femoris m.

Fig. 276

Osteotomy of G. trochanter

If a plate is used for fixation, it should be carefully contoured to the shape of the ilium, using the radiograph of the contralateral, intact ilium, as a guide (Fig. 272). This is important because fracture of the ilium is frequently associated with fracture of the ipsilateral pubis and ischium. However, as the iliac fracture is reduced and its normal contour maintained with the plate, simultaneous reduction of the other fractures usually occurs (Fig. 273).

211

(Wheaton *et al* 1973; Brinker 1975)
Fractures of the acetabulum must be accurately reduced and primary bone union strived for if normal joint function is to be restored. A dorsal approach to the hip is used to expose the fracture (Piermattei & Greeley 1966).

A skin incision is made directly over the hip (Fig. 274). The tensor fascia lata is separated from the biceps femoris to expose the greater trochanter and the gluteal muscles (Figs 275 and 276). A transverse osteotomy of the trochanter is carried out using a saw or osteotome. (N.B. If a lag screw is to be used to re-attach the trochanter, the screw hole should be drilled before the osteotomy is performed). The trochanter is reflected dorsally to expose the joint capsule and dorsal rim of the acetabulum (Fig. 277). An alternative to

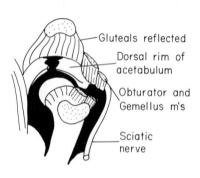

Gluteals reflected

Dorsal rim of acetabulum

Obturator and Gemellus m's

Sciatic nerve

Fig. 277

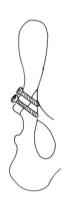

Fig. 278

osteotomy is transection of the tendons of insertion of the gluteal muscles but this is a more traumatic procedure and closure is time consuming. The joint capsule is opened to reveal the femoral head and to allow inspection of the articular surface of the acetabulum. When the fracture involves the caudal part of the joint, it is necessary to expose the body of the ischium; this is achieved after reflection of the gluteal and retraction of the biceps femoris muscles, by severing the insertion of the internal obturator and gemellus muscles close to the trochanteric fossa. These muscles are reflected and used to protect the sciatic nerve to

212

complete the exposure (Fig. 277). After the acetabular fracture has been stabilized the trochanter is re-attached to the femur using either a lag screw, wire tension band or 2 wire sutures.

Oblique fractures of the cranial acetabulum can be stabilized with lag screws (Fig. 278). Transverse fractures of the acetabulum can be stabilized in a number of ways; the application of a plate to the dorsal rim of the acetabulum being the preferred method (Fig. 279). Alternatively fixation can be achieved by inserting 2 screws in the dorsal rim, one on either side of the fracture. A wire figure of eight tension band is then placed around the screw heads to compress the site (Fig. 280). Pins can be used instead of screws (Fig. 281).

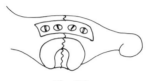

Fig. 279

MULTIPLE PELVIC FRACTURES AND MULTIPLE PELVIC FRACTURES COMPLICATED BY HIND LIMB BONE FRACTURES

Dogs having multiple pelvic fractures with or without hind limb bone fractures are not always good surgical risks in view of the haemorrhage and extensive soft tissue trauma incurred in the accident. However, surgery is undertaken as soon as the animal has recovered from the initial shock and having treated any concommitant injuries to the chest, urinary tract or other soft tissues. The surgical procedures for dogs with multiple fractures are elected to allow pain free movement while subjecting the animal to a minimum of surgical trauma. Both sides of the pelvis may be repaired in one operation if the animal is considered fit enough.

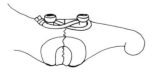

Fig. 280

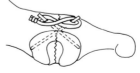

Fig. 281

213

Alternatively repair may be carried out in 2 operations. The management of a typical case is illustrated in Figs 282–284.

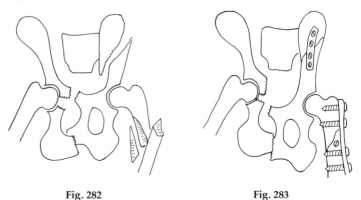

Fig. 282   Fig. 283

Fig. 282. Trace made from the pre-operative radiograph of the pelvis of a 3-year-old Labrador with fractures of the left wing of ilium, left femur, right pubis, ischium, acetabulum and a separation of the right sacro–iliac joint.
Fig. 283. In the first operation the fractures of the left femur and wing of ilium were reduced and plated.

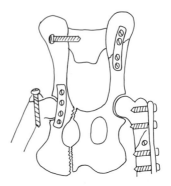

Fig. 284. The second operation was performed 5 days later when the fracture of the right acetabulum was stabilized with a plate and the right sacro–iliac joint with a lag screw.

Surgery of the hip

The hip joint is an enarthrosis and the main movements in the dog are flexion and extension. The anatomy of the joint is illustrated in Figs 285–288. In the skeletally immature dog the main blood supply to the femoral head is derived from

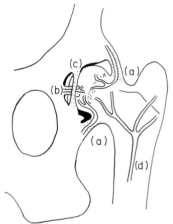

Fig. 285. Ventral view of left hip showing:
(*a*) The joint capsule and the epiphyseal blood vessels
(*b*) The round ligament
(*c*) The trans-acetabular ligament
(*d*) The metaphyseal blood vessels

the epiphyseal vessels associated with the joint capsule while a small amount is derived from vessels running through the round ligament. In the mature dog the femoral head receives an additional blood supply through the metaphyseal vessels but this source becomes available only after fusion of the epiphyseal plate at 8 to 11 months. The soft tissue structures which are of surgical importance are shown in Figs 286–288. Conditions affecting the hip which are amenable to surgical treatment include hip dysplasia, Legge Perthes disease, recurrent or longstanding dislocations of the hip, fractures of the femoral head and fracture of the acetabulum.

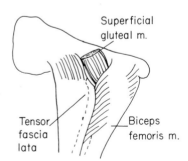

Fig. 286. Superficial lateral muscles of the left hip

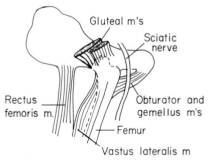

Fig. 287. Deep lateral muscles of the left hip

215

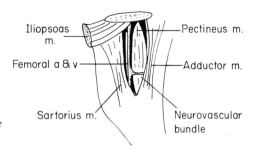

Iliopsoas m.

Femoral a & v

Sartorius m.

Pectineus m.

Adductor m.

Neurovascular bundle

Fig. 288. Muscles of the right hip, medial aspect

SURGICAL APPROACHES TO THE HIP

There are four basic approaches to the hip, cranial, dorsal, caudal and medial. The dorsal approach (page 212, Figs 274–277) is perhaps the simplest and most versatile. The cranial approach is described on page 219, Figs 289–291 and the caudal approach on page 226, Figs 292 & 295.

Hip dysplasia

Hip dysplasia (abnormal development of the hip) is common in most large breeds of dogs, the exception being the Greyhound. Hip dysplasia is a multifactorial disease in which genes, exercise, feeding and other factors play a part (Henricson *et al* 1972).

Dogs are presented for treatment either during the acute growth stage between 4 and 8 months of age, or later in life when secondary osteoarthritic changes have occurred in the hip. History includes, pain on rising, poor exercise tolerance and a 'rolling' gait. On clinical examination the hindquarters are often poorly muscled. Pain, crepitus and excessive laxity may be evident on manipulation of the hips.

Pelvic radiographs are taken under general anaesthesia with the dog on its back, its hind legs fully extended and the stifles inwardly rotated. The radiographic changes in hip dysplasia have been described by Lawson (1973) and Riser (1973). Primary changes seen in the young dog are:

1 Flattening of the femoral head.

2 Lateral displacement of the femoral head with respect to the acetabulum.

3   Luxation or subluxation of the femoral head is seen in severe cases.

These primary changes are followed by degenerative joint disease in older dogs and the associated radiographic changes include:

1   Subchondral erosion of the acetabular margin with osteophyte formation.
2   Flattening of the femoral head due to subchondral eburnation.
3   New bone formation along the articular margin of the femoral head and around the attachments of the joint capsule on the femoral head and trochanteric fossa.

There is no direct correlation between the severity of the clinical signs and the radiographic changes associated with hip dysplasia. Some animals with quite severe radiographic changes live out their lives with little or no evidence of lameness while others with minor radiographic changes may have quite marked episodes of lameness.

The main indications for surgical treatment of hip dysplasia is pain which cannot be relieved by conservative methods such as rest, weight control and the administration of analgesics. Pain associated with hip dysplasia is usually most obvious during the last few months of growth, but once the dog has reached 11 months of age there is usually a spontaneous improvement as the joints stabilize. It is worth advising owners about this and giving the option of surgical treatment if pain and lameness persists after the dog is fully grown.

Methods of surgical treatment include:

1   Resection of the pectineus muscle or its tendon of insertion.
2   Excision arthroplasty.
3   Pelvic osteotomy.
4   Femoral osteotomy.
5   Total hip replacement.

Pectineus myectomy

Considerable attention has been focused on the part played

by the pectineus muscle in the aetiology of hip dysplasia. Bardens & Hardwick (1968) observed that in dogs with hip dysplasia hind leg abduction was limited and the pectineus muscle in such dogs became more prominent and taut as the hip was abducted. Abduction could be increased when the pectineus muscle or its tendon were sectioned. The theory arose that a tight pectineus muscle causes excessive adduction and subluxation of the femoral head. Bardens & Hardwick (1968) claimed that hip dysplasia could be prevented in puppies if the pectineus muscle was sectioned before they reached four weeks of age. This point has been disputed by other workers. However, there have been several reports on the effectiveness of pectineus myectomy or tenotomy in the relief of pain associated with hip dysplasia and this leads to improved locomotion (Wallace 1971; Bowen *et al* 1972; Lust *et al* 1972; Henry 1973; Vaughan *et al* 1975). Why should this procedure relieve pain? Perhaps the pain is due to spasm of the hip muscles and this is relieved when the pectineus muscle is cut, or there is a sudden change in the mechanical forces acting on the upper end of the femur and this stimulates the potential of the deep chondrocytes for proliferation and repair (Nissen 1971). Nevertheless although pectineus myectomy relieves pain the osseous changes associated with hip dysplasia continue unaltered.

TECHNIQUE FOR PECTINEUS MYECTOMY

With the dog in dorsal recumbency and the hind legs fully abducted, the pectineus muscle can be palpated as a prominent, taut band lying directly over the medial aspect of the hip. A skin incision is made over the line of the muscle and the subcutaneous fat is retracted to complete exposure. The muscle is bluntly dissected from the surrounding tissues taking care to avoid the femoral vessels on the cranial aspect, and a neurovascular bundle which crosses the pectineus near its myotendinous junction (Fig. 288). The distal end of the muscle is clamped with artery forceps just proximal to the neurovascular bundle. Using diathery or scissors the muscle is transected close to its origin, and then just proximal to the artery forceps (which prevent retraction following the initial transection). After removal of the muscle belly, care is taken to ensure that all haemorrhage is controlled; minor ooze may be arrested by packing the wound with a swab while the operation is being performed on the other hip. The subcutaneous fat and fascia is co-apted with a continuous catgut suture and the skin with nylon. Post-operative management consists of controlled exercise which, in the case of puppies, should be continued until they are mature. Complications include persistent haematoma formation and recurrence of symptoms due to scar tissue joining the ends of the muscle after inadequate resection.

There is some variation in the results of treatment. Wallace (1971) records a 94% success rate, an improvement being obtained within 24 to 72 hours of surgery. Vaughan *et al* (1975) followed up 100 cases; 80% improved but only 35% had a high standard of recovery, while 20% did not improve or became worse.

Excision arthroplasty

Excision arthroplasty is a salvage procedure and may be used for the treatment of hip dysplasia when conservative methods and/or pectineus myectomy have failed to control the pain. The operation is also indicated in the treatment of Legge Perthes disease and for certain fractures of the femoral head and acetabulum. Duff & Campbell (1977) reviewed the literature on excision arthroplasty and des-cribed the long-term results of the operation. Removal of the femoral head and neck is followed by the development of a pseudo-arthrosis. There is some shortening of the leg, and the range of movement, primarily in extension and abduction, is limited. The gluteal muscles are essential for the support of the joint after excision and ideally an approach (cranial or medial) should be used which avoids damage to these structures. The cranial approach is shown in Figs 274–276 and Figs 289–291.

CRANIAL APPROACH TO THE HIP

The cranial approach to the hip is as in Figs 274–276, the joint is then exposed by blunt dissection within the triangle

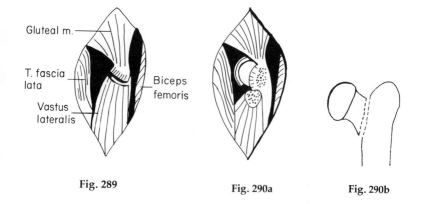

Fig. 289

Fig. 290a

Fig. 290b

bounded by the rectus femoris cranially, the gluteals dorsally and the vastus lateralis caudally (Fig. 289). Such an exposure is limited but can be greatly improved by severing the origin of the vastus lateralis on the femoral neck and reflecting it ventrally (Figs 289, 290). The joint capsule is incised, the round ligament cut and the femoral head dislocated and rotated laterally. The femoral neck is cut flush with the shaft using an osteotome or bone cutters and the head is removed (Fig. 290b). The vastus lateralis is reattached to the gluteals with horizontal mattress sutures of fine catgut.

After removal of the skin sutures, exercise is encouraged. Most dogs regain 'full use' of the leg within three months. The most common cause of failure is inadequate resection of the femoral neck. If bilateral excision is performed a 6–8 week interval should be left between operations.

Pelvic and femoral osteotomies

Pelvic and femoral osteotomies (Brinker 1971; Henry & Wadsworth 1975) have been used in dogs between 4 and 8 months of age to improve stability of the hip. The procedures result in the femoral head being seated more deeply in the acetabulum.

Although the procedures were described in the early 1970s, it is only in recent years that any large series have been undertaken. A lot remains to be learnt about the indi-

220

cations and prognosis although results are promising. The femoral osteotomy known as Intertrochanteric varus osteotomy (Prieur 1982) is technically the easiest to perform. Ideally it is used in dogs with hip dysplasia between 9 and 15 months of age. The normal angle of the femoral neck in relation to the femoral shaft is $146° +$ or $-5°$. If the angle is above this, as in hip dysplasia, the dog is said to have coxa valga. This abnormal angulation contributes to further sub-luxation and instability of the hip. In the intertrochanteric osteotomy a wedge of the proximal femur is removed (Fig. 291a) giving the femoral neck an inclination of approximately 135° (i.e. coxa vara) so that the femoral head tilts further into the acetabulum. The procedure is of benefit not only in young dysplastic dogs but also in older animals with degenerative joint disease because the loading of the damaged articular cartilage is more evenly distributed allowing repair to occur. A special hook plate has been developed (Prieur 1982) (Straumann G. Britain Ltd.) for fixation of the osteotomy (Fig. 291b). The osteotomy heals rapidly and the opposite hip can be operated on 6–8 weeks later if necessary.

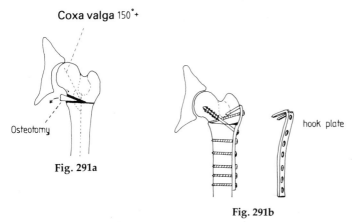

Coxa valga 150° +

Osteotomy

Fig. 291a

hook plate

Fig. 291b

Pelvic osteotomy

This procedure is used in dogs aged 6–12 months with severe hip dysplasia resulting in subluxation of the femoral heads. The aim of surgery is to tilt acetabulum laterally to cover the femoral head more effectively (Figs 291c–e).

221

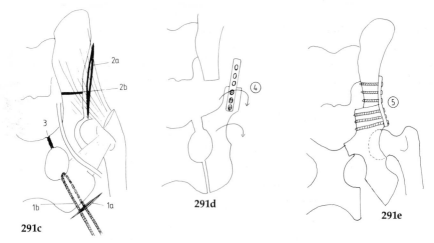

Fig. 291c. (1a) Skin incision over tuber ischii. Subperiotseal elevation of muscle attachments to dorsal and ventral aspects of ischium. Use finger + artery forceps to pass an embryotomy wire through obturator foramen. (1b) Cut ischium with wire. (2a) Skin incision over ventral edge of ilium. Reflect gluteal muscles to expose iliac shaft. Place Hohmann retractors on medial side of ilium to protect sciatic nerve. (2b) Do transverse osteotomy of ileum. Grasp caudal shaft of ilium with bone holders, bend laterally till pubis fractures (3).

Fig. 291d. (4) Attach plate to dorsal rim of ilium then rotate acetabulum laterally to cover femoral head

Fig. 291e. (5) Attach anterior aspect of plate to lateral surface of the shaft of the ilium.

Post-operative management

Restrict dog's exercise until 1 year of age. Bilateral pelvic osteotomy can be done with a 6–8 week interval between each operation.

Total hip replacement

Olmstead *et al* (1981) described the technique for total hip replacement which was used in a series of 132 cases. The procedure gave satisfactory results in 92.5% of cases. Total hip replacement should be used in skeletally mature large breeds of dog with a *painful*, ideally unilateral hip problem which has not responded to other forms of treatment. The main indication is the treatment of hip dysplasia and the procedure can be done bilaterally. The total hip prosthesis

222

consists of a plastic acetabular cup and a stainless steel femoral component (Richards Canine Total Hip Prosthesis, Richards Manufacturing Inc., Memphis, Tennessee, and imported by Alfred Cox Ltd.). The two components are retained in position using polymethyl-methacrylate bone cement. The total hip prosthesis is expensive. The operation must be done under conditions of strict asepsis which cannot be achieved in most practice situations. Special instrumentation and a high degree of technical skill are necessary for correct insertion of the prosthesis. Dislocation of the prosthetic hip can occur at any stage during the first 3 weeks following surgery and exercise must be carefully restricted during this period to prevent this complication arising. Once the joint capsule has healed the hip will remain stable. The more accurate the insertion of the prosthesis, the less the chances of dislocation occurring. Loosening of the implant may occur as a late complication and is invariably due to low grade infection introduced at the time of surgery. A failed total hip replacement can always be converted back to an excision arthroplasty by removal of the implants.

Legge Perthes disease (avascular necrosis of the femoral head) (Spreull 1961; Riser 1963; Ljunggren 1966, 1967; Paatsama 1967, 1969; Lee & Fry 1969; Lee 1970; Smith 1971)

Legge Perthes disease is a disease of young dogs between 3 and 9 months of age. The small breeds, in particular the Terriers, are usually affected. There is interference with the blood supply to the femoral head which results in avascular necrosis. The factors which interfere with the blood supply are not completely understood but several reasons have been postulated and are listed below.

1   Trauma to the epiphyseal blood vessels (Fig. 285) resulting in thrombosis.

2   Imbalance of sex hormones. Legge Perthes disease has been reproduced experimentally by the administration of high levels of oestrogen or androgen. The result is premature closure of the proximal epiphyseal plate of the femur and a disturbance in the circulation (Ljunggren 1967).

3 Genetic factors. There is evidence for a genetic pre–disposition as a high incidence of the disease follows certain breed lines. Pidduck and Webber (1978), in an analysis of the pedigrees of Toy Poodles affected with Legge Perthes disease from one kennel obtained results consistent with the hypothesis that Perthes disease is caused by homo–zygosity for an autosomal recessive gene.

The histological and radiographic changes associated with Legge Perthes disease have been described (Lee 1970).

The initial change is ischaemic necrosis of the femoral head. There may be little clinical evidence of lameness or radiological abnormality at this stage. Continued weight bearing causes trabecular fragmentation, deformity and cavitation and a radiograph reveals uneven femoral head density with deformity.

Next, highly vascular granulation tissue penetrates the growth plate and results in revascularization and replace-ment of the dead tissues by a process of 'creeping substi-tution'. The removal of bone and deposition of foci of closely trabeculated bone and areas of fibrous tissue gives the femoral head an uneven density on radiographic examination.

Although the femoral head is revascularized and re-modelled, deformity inevitably persists and this is associa-ted with osteophytic proliferation around the femoral neck and acetabular rim.

The clinical signs are a gradual onset of unilateral or bilateral hind leg lameness over a period of 3–4 months. The degree of lameness becomes gradually worse until the dog only uses the leg intermittently or carries it. There is obvious muscle wasting and pain on manipulation of the hip, par-ticularly when it is abducted. This degree of lameness remains static for a further 1 or 2 months and then there is gradual improvement.

Excision arthroplasty is considered to be the best method of treating most cases of Legge Perthes disease (Ljunggren 1966). In a group of 36 cases treated in this way, 30 regained good use of the affected leg. By comparison, of 62 cases treated by conservative methods, only 15 regained use of the leg and a longer period of convalescence was required.

Conservative treatment involves complete rest during the first 3 months after the onset of lameness, followed by the encouragement of exercise and passive manipulation of the hip to prevent muscle atrophy and help mould the head of the femur to the shape of the acetabulum and limit the degree of deformity.

Dislocation of the hip

Dislocation of the hip is a common injury in the dog. Affected animals are usually over one year of age. The femoral head is dislocated in a craniodorsal direction in 85–90% of cases, cranioventral in 2–3% of cases, while caudoventral and caudodorsal dislocations are rare.

In craniodorsal dislocations the dog carries the leg semi-flexed and adducted under the body. If both hind legs are extended and their length compared, then the affected leg will appear shorter and the distance between the greater trochanter and tuber ischii will be greater than on the normal side. Radiographs should be taken of the hips to confirm the diagnosis and eliminate the presence of fractures.

Closed reduction should be attempted within 48 hours. The dog is anaesthetized and placed on its side with the dislocated hip uppermost. A towel is placed under the leg and used to anchor it to the edge of the table or alternatively, it is held by an assistant. Traction is exerted on the limb in a caudal direction and at the same time it is slightly abducted so that the femoral head is lifted over the rim of the acetabulum. At the same time thumb pressure is applied to the greater trochanter to stop the femoral head slipping ventrally around the rim of the acetabulum. If reduction is successful the femoral head should be forced down into the acetabulum to express any blood clot and the joint flexed and extended several times to check the stability of the reduction. If the joint tends to redislocate when the leg is extended the limb is strapped with the stifle and hock in flexion for three to five days (Fig. 33f).

Recurrent or longstanding (up to two months) dislocations require open reduction and fixation. Knowles *et al* (1953) were the first to describe a satisfactory method of fixation by replacing the ligamentum teres with a strip of fascia which was anchored in the acetabular fossa by a toggle pin. Similar techniques have been described by Lawson (1965) and Denny & Minter (1973) using braided nylon as a substitute for the ligament, by Leonard (1971) employing stainless steel wire or a heavy plastic suture, and by Zakiewicz (1967) using skin.

Stabilization of the hip using a toggle pin and a braided nylon round ligament prosthesis

The majority of hip dislocations occur in a craniodorsal direction and consequently the gemellus and obturator muscles which insert on the caudal aspect of the proximal femur, are often torn or stretched over the acetabulum thus providing a ready made approach (Fig. 292).

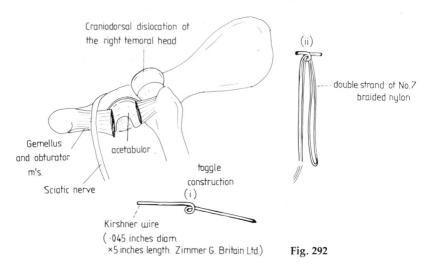

Fig. 292

Technique

A skin incision is made directly over the greater trochanter and continued distally over the femur to the midshaft region (Fig. 293). The fascia lata is separated from the biceps femoris muscle using scissors (Fig. 293). The biceps

226

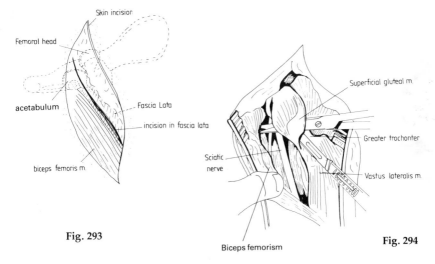

Fig. 293

Biceps femorism

Fig. 294

femoris is retracted to reveal the greater trochanter. The sciatic nerve is identified caudal to the femoral shaft in the loose fascia between the biceps femoris and the semi-membranosus muscle. The path of the nerve is traced proximally around the hip (Fig. 294). The nerve is carefully protected while exposure of the acetabulum is completed from the caudal aspect. The insertion of the superficial gluteal muscle is transected and the caudal muscles of the hip (obturator and gemelli) if not already ruptured, are transected close to their insertion on the proximal femur (Fig. 295a). These muscles are reflected and the dislocated

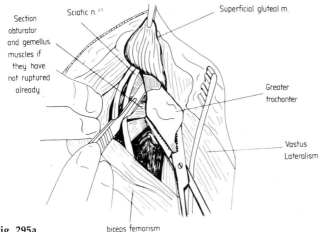

Fig. 295a

biceps femorism

femoral head is retracted cranial to the acetabulum with bone holding forceps applied to the proximal femoral shaft. Torn joint capsule is trimmed back and the acetabulum is cleared of haematoma or granulation tissue. When a pseudoarthrosis has formed in a long standing dislocation, thickened joint capsule must be removed and adhesions between the femoral head and dorsal rim of the acetabulum broken down before reduction of the dislocation can be achieved.

Once the acetabulum has been debrided, a tunnel is drilled through the acetabular fossa using a 3/16ths drill bit (Fig. 295b). Artery forceps are used to guide the toggle into the tunnel then the blunt end of the 7/64ths drill bit is used to push the toggle completely through the acetabulum. Traction is applied to the braided nylon round ligament prosthesis to ensure that the toggle rotates and engages firmly on the medial side of the acetabulum. (Fig. 295b).

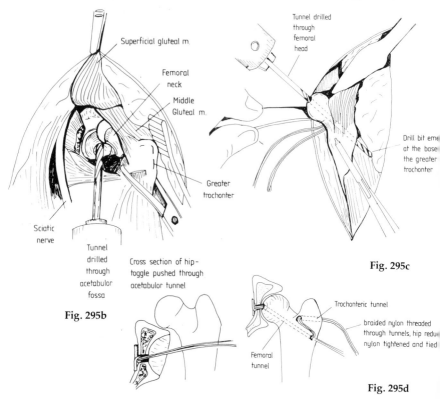

Superficial gluteal m.

Femoral neck

Middle Gluteal m.

Greater trochanter

Sciatic nerve

Tunnel drilled through acetabular fossa

Cross section of hip-toggle pushed through acetabular tunnel

Fig. 295b

Tunnel drilled through femoral head

Drill bit eme at the base the greater trochanter

Fig. 295c

Trochonteric tunnel

braided nylon threaded through tunnels, hip redu nylon tightened and tied

Femoral tunnel

Fig. 295d

228

The femoral head is rotated in a caudolateral direction. The blade of a Hohmann retractor is inserted between the caudal border of the gluteal muscles and the femoral neck. The retractor is used to elevate the femoral head out of the incision and remnants of the round ligament are removed. A second Hohmann retractor may be necessary to depress the biceps femoris muscle while a tunnel is drilled using a 7/64ths bit from the fovea capitis through the femoral head and neck to emerge just ventral to the greater trochanter (Figs 295c,d). A second tunnel is drilled through the greater trochanter (Fig. 295d). Wire loops are placed through both tunnels. The braided nylon is drawn through the femoral tunnel using a loop. Traction is maintained on the nylon while the dislocation is reduced. Half the nylon is drawn through the trochanteric tunnel using the remaining wire loop and the free ends of the prosthesis are tightly tied. Reduction and stability of the hip should be checked before cutting off the excess nylon. Once reduction is complete, the obturator and gemellus muscle are no longer easily accessible and are left unsutured. The transected superficial gluteal muscle is repaired using horizontal mattress sutures of fine monofilament nylon. The fascia lata and biceps femoris, the subcutaneous fascia and skin are coapted in layers in routine fashion.

Post–operative care
The leg is strapped in flexion for 5 days and skin sutures are generally removed after 8 days. Exercise is severely restricted for 4 weeks post–operatively. The progress is usually good and 84% of cases will regain full limb function. In the remainder varying degrees of lameness persist.

Post–operative complications
1 Re–dislocation with rupture of the braided nylon round ligament prosthesis. Factors predisposing to premature breakage of the prosthesis include overactivity in the recovery period, hip dysplasia and muscle contraction in longstanding dislocations. The hip joint may be salvaged by excision of the femoral head.
2 If dislocation occurs in an immature dog before closure

of the proximal femoral growth plate, then rupture of the joint capsule may lead to ischaemic necrosis of the femoral head. When this complication arises after the hip toggle procedure, excision arthroplasty should be carried out.

3   Osteoarthritis—this is a possible complication of any joint injury.

Fractures of the femoral head and neck

Fractures of the femoral head and capital epiphysis are common in young dogs. When the fracture occurs within the joint capsule (intracapsular) the blood supply to the femoral head is disrupted and avascular necrosis may ensue. A further complication is non-union due to in-adequate reduction and poor stabilization. For these reasons, excision of the femoral head and neck is often the preferred method of treatment. However, open reduction and rigid fixation of the fracture by interfragmental com-pression using a lag screw (Fig. 296) gives good results

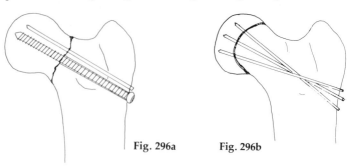

Fig. 296a   Fig. 296b

provided surgery is carried out soon after the accident, preferably within 48 hours (Hulse *et al* 1974). The fracture is exposed using the anterior or dorsal approach. Initial fixation of the fracture is achieved with a Kirschner wire which prevents rotation as the lag screw is inserted. In young dogs with separation or fracture separation of the capital femoral epiphysis 3 Kirschner wires are used for fixation (Fig. 296b). Lysis of the dorsal aspect of the femoral neck is often seen on follow up radiographs taken 4–6 weeks after surgery. This is probably due to a local dis-turbance in blood supply. The zone subsequently revas-cularizes and remodels.

230

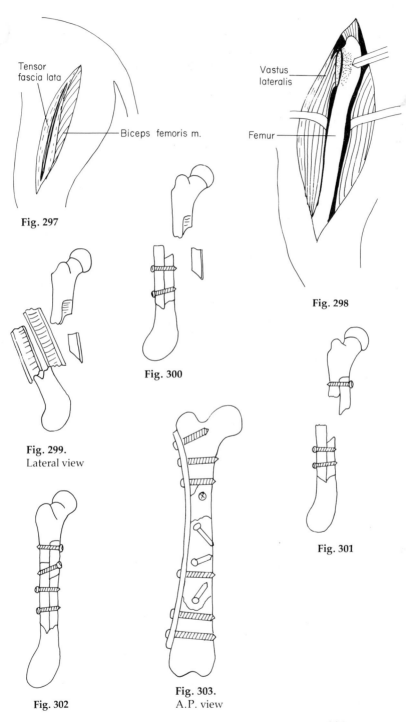

Tensor fascia lata

Biceps femoris m.

Fig. 297

Vastus lateralis

Femur

Fig. 298

Fig. 299.
Lateral view

Fig. 300

Fig. 301

Fig. 302

Fig. 303.
A.P. view

Fracture of the capital epiphysis is sometimes accompanied by separation of the greater trochanter (Denny 1971). The latter may be missed on an A.P. radiograph of the hips but should be obvious on a lateral view. The trochanteric separation provides a ready-made dorsal approach for either excision or lag screw fixation of the femoral head. The trochanter is then re-attached with a lag screw, or wire tension band.

Fractures of the acetabulum

These have already been described under pelvic fractures (see page 212).

Fractures of the shaft of the femur

Fractures of the femur are common. Simple transverse fractures of the shaft in young dogs are best treated by intramedullar fixation (see page 44, Figs 35–38), while plate and screw fixation is used for comminuted and oblique fractures especially in large dogs. The plate is usually applied to the lateral aspect of the shaft.

The femur is exposed by a lateral skin incision extending from the greater trochanter to the stifle. The attachment between the tensor fascia lata and the biceps femoris is cut and blunt dissection between the vastus lateralis and biceps femoris will reveal the femoral shaft (Figs 297 and 298). The incision can be extended into the joint capsule of the stifle to complete exposure of the distal femur as necessary. Exposure of the proximal shaft is achieved by subperiosteal elevation and cranial reflection of the origin of the vastus lateralis muscle (Fig. 298).

Figs 299–303 illustrate the stages in the repair of a comminuted fracture of the femur using lag screws and a plate. Soft tissue attachments to the fragments are retained where possible. Ideally lag screws are inserted in a craniocaudal or caudocranial direction so that they do not interfere with the application of a plate to the lateral surface of the femur. However, due to the plane of the fracture it is sometimes necessary to place the lag screws in a lateromedial direction. Under these circumstances temporary reduction of the fragments can be achieved with a cerclage wire (Fig. 304). The plate is applied and screws inserted through the plate are used to lag the fragments together (Fig. 304). The cerclage wire is removed before the screws are finally tightened.

Segmental fractures of the femur (Fig. 305) are sometimes encountered. Although these may be stabilized with an intramedullary pin there is a risk of rotation at one or other of the fracture sites. The dynamic compression plate is an ideal method of fixation and permits axial compression of both fractures sites (Fig. 306).

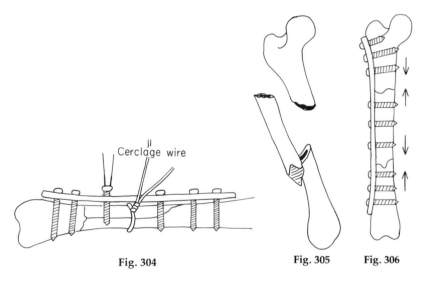

Cerclage wire

Fig. 304   Fig. 305   Fig. 306

The treatment of femoral shaft fractures in puppies deserves a short mention. An intramedullary pin can be used for fixation in most instances. However reduction should be undertaken with a minimum of soft tissue trauma as a common complication of the fracture is the formation of adhesions between the quadriceps and femur which result in rigid extension of the stifle (see p. 235).

If a pin is broken off flush below the level of the greater trochanter, rapid longitudinal growth of the femur in the puppy usually results in the pin becoming sealed within the medullary cavity and prevents its retrieval. Consequently if removal of an intramedullary pin is contemplated radiographs should always be taken to check its position.

Supracondylar fractures of the femur

Supracondylar fractures of the femur are usually seen in animals between 3 and 10 months of age but can also occur in adult animals. The fracture occurs wholly or partially through the growth plate. There is pain and crepitus on manipulation but gross instability is not always a feature and such fractures can sometimes be missed in a cursory examination. The fracture however is obvious on radiographic examination (Fig. 307).

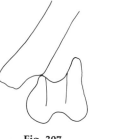

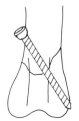

Fig. 307   Fig. 308

Treatment in dogs 7 months of age or over is by open reduction and fixation with a lag screw (Fig. 308) (Knight 1956; Hinko 1974). The fracture involves the stifle joint and the advantage of screw fixation is that optimal stability is provided and the fracture should heal with minimal callus formation. The fracture is exposed through a lateral para-patellar skin incision, the lateral aspect of the joint capsule is incised and the patella if it has not already been displaced is reflected to reveal the fracture site. Reduction is not always easy, an ideal pair of bone holding forceps for gripping the distal epiphysis of the femur is shown in ʁ g. 309. These forceps are also useful to maintain reduction of the fracture (Fig. 310) while the lag screw is inserted.

Other methods of fixation include cross pinning (Fig. 311) (Sumner Smith & Dingwall 1973), Rush pins (Fig. 43), 3-hole plate (Fig. 312) (Hickman 1964) or wire suture (Fig. 313)

234

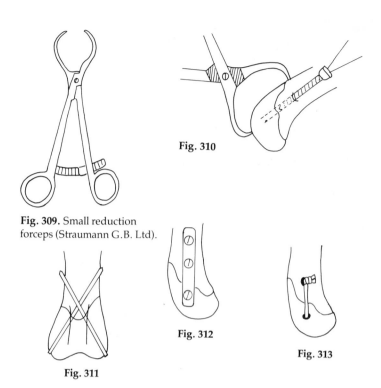

Fig. 309. Small reduction forceps (Straumann G.B. Ltd).

Fig. 310

Fig. 311

Fig. 312

Fig. 313

in miniature dogs. Cross pinning or Rush pins are recommended for fixation in pups under 6 months of age because these methods cause minimal disturbance in longitudinal growth. The other methods mentioned here will cause premature closure of the growth plate unless the implant is removed within 3–4 weeks.

Failure to treat a supracondylar fracture by internal fixation usually results in ankylosis of the stifle joint. Because the condyles rotate caudally, the distal shaft of the femur is displaced anteriorly and the patella becomes involved in a mass of callus at the fracture site.

Fracture of a single condyle (Fig. 314a) or both condyles of the distal femur ('T' fracture, Fig. 314c) are rare. Lag screws are used for fixation as in Fig. 314b and 314d.

Contracture of the quadriceps femoris muscles
(Vaughan 1979)

Quadriceps contracture can occur as a congenital deformity

or a complication of femoral shaft fractures in puppies. The latter is seen most frequently. Splints or casts which fit tightly round the mid–thigh may cause muscle ischaemia leading to contracture. Alternatively internal fixation of shaft fractures may be followed by adhesion of the quadriceps to the fracture site.

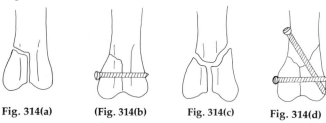

Fig. 314(a)   (Fig. 314(b)   Fig. 314(c)   Fig. 314(d)

The clinical features of quadriceps contracture are:
1   Rigid extension of the stifle.
2   Hyperextension of the hock.
3   The foot tends to be dragged, giving excoriation of the dorsum.
4   Quadriceps become fibrous and taut.
   A lateral radiograph of the stifle shows the patella riding high in the femoral trochlea. Congenital contracture leads to genu recurvatum, with deformity of the distal femur, proximal tibia and a patella riding some distance proximal to the trochlea (Fig. 315).

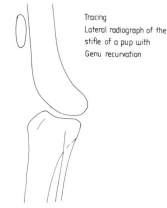

Tracing
Lateral radiograph of the
stifle of a pup with
Genu recurvation

Fig. 315

Treatment
If adhesions have formed between the quadriceps and femur, then surgical release and vigorous physiotherapy

236

may improve the range of stifle movement. Quadriceps-plasty—section of each of the quadriceps muscles—is used for congenital or ischaemic contractures. The leg is then maintained in semi–flexion with a splint or bandage for 2 weeks to encourage lengthening of the quadriceps during the healing process and an improved leg posture.

The prognosis is not good however and a recurrence of contracture frequently occurs despite these procedures.

Rupture of the gracilis muscle (Bateman 1960; Sanders 1962; Bateman 1964; Davis 1967; Vaughan 1969; Hickman 1975)

Rupture of the gracilis muscle is seen in the racing Greyhound. The right hind leg is most frequently affected and injury to the muscle is usually accompanied by haematoma formation. Tears of the muscle occur in a number of positions, through the belly of the muscle, the musculo-tendinous junction and at the conjoined tendon of insertion with the sartorius and semitendinosis muscle. The caudal border of the muscle is most frequently involved.

Hickman (1975) recommends that in recent cases treatment should be directed towards a radical surgical repair rather than conservative treatment (cold applications, pressure bandages and aspiration to limit the size of the haematoma). Surgical exposure of the medial aspect of the thigh allows inspection of the damaged tissues. The haematoma can be drained and haemorrhage controlled but more important accurate anatomical reconstruction of the torn muscle may be carried out using a series of mattress sutures. Consequently, after repair the torn muscles should heal with a minimum of fibrous tissue formation and not impede the animal's future racing potential.

Conservative treatment invariably leads to excessive fibrous tissue formation which may require surgical release (Bateman 1964) to improve the dog's action.

Contracture of the gracilis muscle in the alsatian (Vaughan 1979)

Contracture of the Gracilis muscle in Alsatians causes a

characteristic alteration in gait. The condition has been recorded in dogs between 3 and 7 years of age and affected animals have generally led extremely active lives. Gait changes suddenly and deteriorates over a period of 6 weeks and then remains static. When walking, the affected leg is raised in a jerky fashion with the hock hyperflexed and rotated outwards while the foot is turned inwards. The Gracilis muscle can be palpated as a taut band on the medial aspect of the thigh.

Section of the Gracilis tendon gives immediate relief but recurrence of the gait defect usually occurs 3–5 months after surgery. Dogs continue to lead an active life despite the condition. In the Alsatian, contracture involves the tendon of insertion of the Gracilis, unlike the Greyhound where the muscle belly is affected.

SURGERY OF THE STIFLE JOINT

The canine stifle is a complex joint and is illustrated in Figs 316–318. Primary motion within the joint is hingelike.

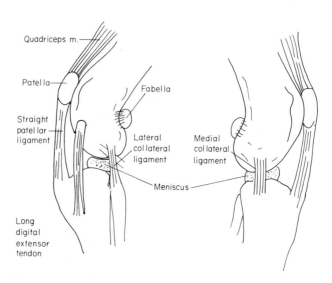

Fig. 316. Lateral view of stifle   **Fig. 317.** Medial view of stifle

238

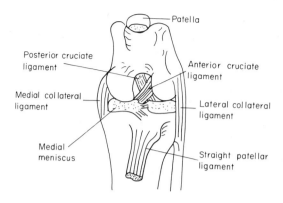

Fig. 318. Anterior view of stifle

Figs 316–318 reproduced by permission of Miller M.E. (1952). *Guide to the Dissection of the Dg.* 3rd Ed. Edwards Brothers. Michigan.

Traumatic injuries of the stifle include:

1   Supracondylar and condylar fractures of the femur (see page 234, Figs 307–315).

2   Fractures of the patella or avulsion of the straight patellar ligament.

3   Avulsion of the tibial tuberosity.

4   Avulsion of the tibial tuberosity with separation or fracture of the proximal epiphysis of the tibia.

5   Avulsion of the tendon of origin of the long digital extensor muscle.

6   Rupture of the anterior cruciate ligament and meniscal injuries.

7   Rupture of the posterior cruciate ligament.

8   Rupture of a collateral ligament.

9   Dislocation of the stifle.

10   Traumatic dislocation of the patella.

Diseases of the stifle joint include:

1   Congenital dislocation of the patella.

2   Osteochondritis dissecans of the femoral condyles.

3   Degenerative joint disease secondary to stifle injuries.

4   Osteosarcoma—the distal femur or the proximal tibia are common sites for primary osteosarcoma.

Fractures of the patella, or avulsion of the straight patellar ligament (Denny 1975; Betts & Walker 1975)

Fracture of the patella is rare. The injury is caused by direct violence and results in a variety of fractures, transverse, longitudinal or comminuted. Transverse fracture of the patella (Fig. 319) or an avulsion of the straight patellar ligament (Fig. 320) results in inability to fully extend the stifle. On palpation the straight patellar ligament feels slack

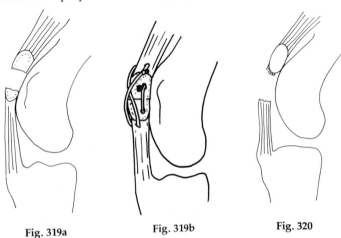

Fig. 319a   Fig. 319b   Fig. 320

and the patella rides 'high' in the trochlea. A lateral radiograph of the stifle will confirm the diagnosis. Another useful radiographic view to demonstrate the number of fragments is a sky-line view of the patella (Figs 321 and 322). A transverse fracture is repaired by the use of a wire suture and wire tension band (Fig. 319b).

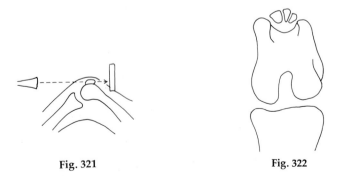

Fig. 321   Fig. 322

240

If avulsion of the straight patellar ligament has occurred, small fragments of bone are removed from the end of the ligament. A Bunnel tendon suture of wire is inserted (Fig. 323) and used to reattach the ligament to the patella. The wire is anchored to the patella through a transverse tunnel (Figs 323 and 324). Longitudinal fractures of the patella can be stabilized with a lag screw (Fig. 325).

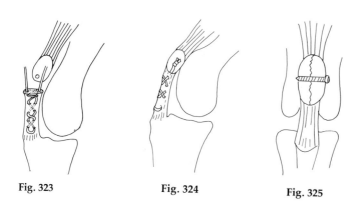

Fig. 323 Fig. 324 Fig. 325

Comminuted fractures of the patella are a problem, if the fragments are large enough they may be screwed or wired together. In some cases this is a technical impossibility and under these circumstances patellectomy is performed. This could be followed by a homogenous patella transplant. This operation has been successfully undertaken in experimental dogs (Vaughan & Formston 1973).

Avulsion of the tibial tuberosity (Dingwall & Sumner-Smith 1971; Pettit & Slatter 1973; Denny 1975; Withrow *et al* 1976)

Fractures of the tibial tuberosity (Fig. 326) are avulsion fractures. The fragment is distracted by the pull of the quadriceps on the patella and straight patella ligament. The fracture is usually associated with a fall or jumping and is seen in dogs between 4 and 8 months of age. Treatment of the fracture is by open reduction and fixation using either Kirschner wires and a wire tension band (Figs 75–77) or a lag screw plus tension band wire (Fig. 327). The prognosis is usually good and the implants can be left *in situ*.

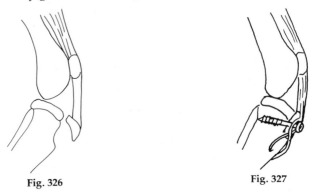

Fig. 326   Fig. 327

Avulsion of the tibial tuberosity and fracture of separation of the proximal epiphysis of the tibia

Fracture through the proximal growth plate of the tibia is seen in immature dogs occasionally and results in caudal displacement of the epiphysis (Fig. 328). Treatment is by open reduction and fixation is achieved by 2 transfixion pins

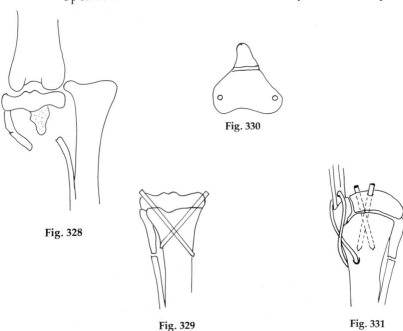

Fig. 330

Fig. 328

Fig. 329   Fig. 331

242

inserted down through the medial and lateral side of the proximal tibial epiphysis into the metaphysis (Fig. 329 and 330). The tibial tuberosity is then stabilized with a wire tension band (Fig. 331).

Avulsion of the tendon of origin of the long digital extensor muscle (Denny & Minter 1973; Pond 1973)

The long digital extensor muscle arises on the lateral condyle of the distal femur, crosses the femorotibial joint and passes beneath the anterior tibial muscle (Fig. 316). Avulsion of the tendon of origin is occasionally encountered in young dogs (average age of recorded cases is 6 months).

There is a sudden onset of lameness, the leg is carried and there is swelling, pain but no instability evident on manipulation of the stifle. After the acute stage has subsided, mild lameness with slight discomfort on palpation persists. A lateral radiograph of the stifle will reveal a radiolucent defect in the anterior aspect of the distal femoral epiphysis with a small fragment of calcified material lying in the joint ventral to the defect (Fig. 332). Other conditions to consider

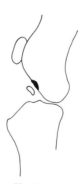

Fig. 332

in the differential diagnosis are osteochondritis dissecans and avulsion of the anterior cruciate ligament. The latter however, will result in joint instability.

An exploratory arthrotomy will confirm the diagnosis and the fragment of bone is removed (it is possible to provide a new site of origin for the long digital extensor tendon by suturing it to the lateral collateral ligament. Pond (1973) recommends that the avulsed fragment is retained in its normal position with a lag screw.

Cruciate ligament rupture

Cruciate ligament rupture is common and can be encountered in any breed of dog. In 1973, the author reviewed a series of 159 cases with rupture of the anterior cruciate ligament. 28 breeds were affected and the condition was seen most frequently in the Poodle and the Labrador. No cases were seen in dogs under a year of age and the peak incidence was at 6 years with a lesser peak at 2 years. In the younger dog there was usually a sudden onset of lameness during exercise or through the dog catching its leg in a fence or other obstacle. In the older dogs lameness was often more insidious in onset and perhaps this is related to degenerative changes in the ligament before rupture. Bilateral rupture tended to be seen in this group of animals especially those that were overweight. However, in none of the bilateral cases had the ruptures occurred simultaneously.

The ligament most commonly affected is the anterior cruciate ligament. Sometimes there is concurrent rupture of the posterior cruciate ligament resulting in marked instability. However, rupture of the posterior cruciate ligament alone is uncommon. The function of the anterior cruciate ligament is to prevent anterior displacement of the tibia in relation to the femur. The clinical signs associated with rupture have been described (Carlin 1926; Brook 1952; Paatsama 1952; Hickman 1954; Leonard 1971). Following rupture of the anterior cruciate ligament the leg is carried with the stifle slightly flexed. There is usually little swelling of the joint and passive manipulation is seldom resented. After 7–10 days the dog begins to use the leg when walking but at rest stands with the toe just touching the ground. Atrophy of the thigh muscles is usually evident at this stage and when walking a clicking sound may be heard due to the femoral condyles slipping in and out of their normal

244

position on the menisci. Diagnosis of rupture of the anterior cruciate ligament is confirmed by demonstration of an anterior draw sign (Fig. 333). The dog is positioned on its

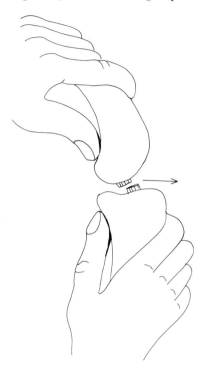

Fig. 333

side with the affected leg uppermost, the shaft of the femur is firmly fixed in one hand with the thumb placed behind the femoral condyle. The proximal shaft of the tibia is grasped in the other hand with the thumb behind the tibia. If the anterior cruciate ligament is ruptured it should be possible to move the tibia forward in relation to the femoral condyles. This is known as the anterior draw sign. Normally there is no movement in this plane. If there is any doubt about the stability of the joint due to muscle spasm or pain, the anterior draw movement should be tested after the administration of a general anaesthetic.

Instability of the stifle is followed by degenerative joint disease. Periarticular osteophytes develop and on a radiograph these are most obvious on the poles of the patella, the fabellae, the edges of the trochlea and the articular margins of the tibia. The weight of the dog has a marked influence on the development of the osteophytic reaction (Heffron 1976). Hence minimal osteophytic reactions are seen in the small breeds of dog but early and rapid development of osteophytes occur in the heavy breeds. Reduction in the use of the limb by strict rest slows the rate of osteophyte formation (Campbell 1977). The joint becomes thickened particularly on the medial aspect as a result of periarticular fibrosis and restabilization may occur in 6–8 weeks. During this time lameness improves but although it may apparently resolve it tends to recur after vigorous exercise.

Small dogs usually respond to conservative treatment consisting of strict rest for at least 6 weeks. No analgesics or corticosteroids are necessary during this period. In the larger breeds especially working dogs, it is generally agreed that some form of surgical stabilization should be performed. Various techniques have been employed, these were reviewed by Knecht 1976. Paatsama (1952) used fascia lata to replace the ligament; other modifications of this technique are replacement with skin (Gibbens 1957; Vaughan 1963; Vaughan & Bowden 1964), with synthetic materials (Johnson 1960; Emery & Rostrup 1960; Ormrod 1963; Singleton 1963; Vaughan 1963; Vaughan & Bowden 1964; Singleton 1969a; Gupta & Brinker 1969), with skin and monofilament nylon (Pond & Campbell 1972), and with the tendon of the peroneus longus muscle (Rathor 1960). Other methods include stabilization of the joint by means of segment of the patella and its ligament (Strande 1966), translocation of the tendon of the long digital extensor muscle (Hohn & Miller, 1967; Lewis 1974), and posterior capsulorrhaphy (Hohn & Newton, personal communication). More recently, carbon fibre has been used for cruciate ligament replacement (Denny & Goodship 1980). However, the major advance in treatment since Paatsama's original work has been the development of the 'over the top' technique (Arnoczky et al 1979) in which the anterior cruciate is replaced with part of the patellar ligament complex.

246

Technique for replacement of the anterior cruciate ligament with a braided nylon prosthesis Singleton (1969a) (Fig. 334)

The operation is performed with the dog lying on its back. A lateral parapatellar skin incision is made (Fig. 335a). The

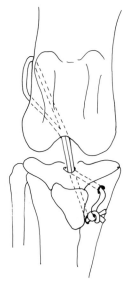

Fig. 334

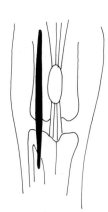

Fig. 335(a)

lateral aspect of the joint capsule is incised longitudinally and the patella dislocated medially to expose the trochlea. The stifle is flexed to allow inspection of the torn ends of the anterior cruciate ligament and the menisci. (A nutrient artery crosses the anterior aspect of the joint and those uninitiated in cruciate surgery may mistake this for a remnant of the ligament). If the medial meniscus is obviously torn or displaced into the anterior aspect of the joint then meniscectomy is carried out. Osteophytes in and around the trochlea are trimmed off with a scalpel. The patella should also be inspected for osteophytes and in most dogs it is possible to completely reflect the patella to expose

247

its articular surface. Two tunnels are drilled starting from the lateral condyle of the femur, these merge together in the intercondyloid fossa at the origin of the anterior cruciate ligament (Figs 335b,c). Two tunnels which diverge from the point of insertion of the ligament on the tibial plateau are drilled to emerge on the medial aspect of the tibial crest (Fig. 335c).

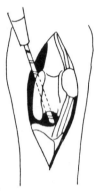 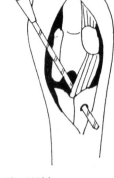

Fig. 335(b)   **Fig. 335(c)**

Wire loops are used to thread the braided nylon prosthesis through the femoral and tibial tunnels. The patella is reduced, the stifle fully extended and the ends of the nylon tied tightly leaving a knot on the medial aspect of the tibia. (No. 7 braided nylon is used, two strands cross the joint in a small dog and up to 16 are used in a large dog). On occasions the tunnels in the tibia may be drilled too close together and the bone between them collapses. The situation can be salvaged by drilling a further tunnel transversely through the tibial crest to allow the end of the prosthesis to be tied off.

The joint is flushed out with normal saline and penicillin before the joint capsule is closed with simple interrupted sutures of monofilament nylon. Subsequent wound closure is routine. A support bandage is applied for 5 days and antibiotic cover is given during this period. Most dogs begin to use the affected leg again within 10 days to 3 weeks. Exercise should be severely restricted for 2 months following surgery.

The main advantages of the technique are the relative speed and ease of operation and stability of the joint is restored immediately. Subsequently wear and tear undoubtedly leads to stretching or fragmentation of the prosthesis but by that stage the joint has been stabilized by periarticular fibrosis.

Failures are usually due to dirty surgical technique or inadequate size of prosthesis. Braided nylon when used under sterile conditions does not provoke a foreign body reaction and such reactions are invariably due to low grade infection.

Arnoczky's 'over the top' technique for anterior cruciate ligament replacement

The original 'over the top' procedure was described by Arnoczky *et al* in 1979. A graft consisting of the medial third of the straight patellar ligament, a wedge of the patella and fascia lata was prepared and drawn through the stifle joint over the remnants of the anterior cruciate ligament. The graft was tightened and the free end sutured to the lateral condyle of the femur (Fig. 336a, b and c). The procedure is the most biologically sound method of cruciate ligament replacement to have been described in recent years. The normal anatomy and orientation of the anterior cruciate ligament is duplicated, and it was demonstrated in experimental dogs that the graft was revascularized from the caudal aspect of the joint and developed into a functional ligament. The procedure immediately restores joint stability and has proved an excellent method for treating anterior cruciate ligament rupture in large and giant breeds of dog. Two variations on the original procedure are presented here:

1 'Over the Top' using fascia lata as a graft.
2 'Over the Top' using the middle third of the straight patella ligament.

Over the top using fascia lata as a graft

The technique can be used in dogs of any size. The dog is

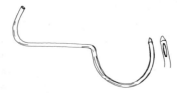

Fig. 336(a)

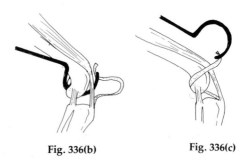

Fig. 336(b)   **Fig. 336(c)**

placed on its back for surgery. A lateral parapatellar skin incision is made (Fig. 335a) and extended through subcutaneous fascia and fat. Two parallel incisions are made from the tibial crest and extended proximally on the lateral side of the joint to produce a graft consisting of the lateral third of the straight patella ligament and fascia lata

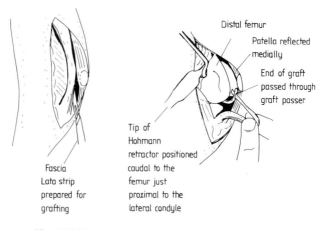

Fascia
Lata strip
prepared for
grafting

Tip of
Hohmann
retractor positioned
caudal to the
femur just
proximal to the
lateral condyle

Distal femur

Patella reflected
medially

End of graft
passed through
graft passer

Fig. 336(d)   **Fig. 336(e)**

250

(see Fig. 336d). The graft is reflected ventrally but its distal attachment to the tibial crest is retained. A lateral parapatellar arthrotomy incision is then made and the patella is reflected medially (Fig. 336e). Management of osteophytes or torn medial meniscus is as already described on page 247. The lateral condyle of the femur is exposed by retracting the joint capsule with a Hohmann retractor (Fig. 336e) (Straumann Great Britain Ltd). The tip of the retractor is introduced behind the femur just proximal to the lateral fabella. The ligamentous attachments between the fabella and the femur are severed with a scalpel to allow access to the caudal joint space. A graft passer (see Fig. 336a) is introduced through this incision into the intercondylar fossa and out into the cranial joint space (Fig. 336e). The free end of the graft is passed through the 'eye' of the graft passer and the instrument is used to draw the graft through the joint over the top of the remnants of the original anterior cruciate ligament and out over the lateral fabella (Fig. 336f). The patella is returned to its normal position, the graft is pulled tight and the free end sutured to the periosteum of the lateral condyle (Fig. 336g) of the femur using mono- filament nylon or fine braided wire sutures. The same suture material is used to close the joint capsule and the rest of the wound closure is routine. A support bandage is applied for 5 days and skin sutures are removed at 10 days. Exercise is severely restricted for 6 weeks and then gradu- ally increased. Full limb function should be regained within 3 months.

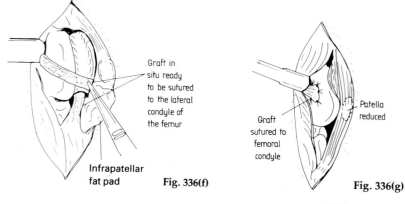

Graft in situ ready to be sutured to the lateral condyle of the femur

Infrapatellar fat pad

Fig. 336(f)

Graft sutured to femoral condyle

Patella reduced

Fig. 336(g)

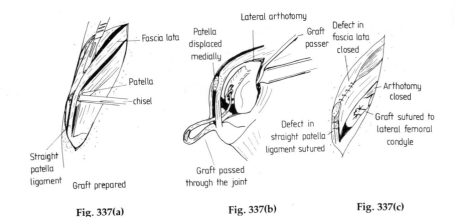

Straight patella ligament   Graft prepared

Fascia lata

Patella

chisel

Patella displaced medially

Lateral arthotomy

Graft passer

Defect in fascia lata closed

Defect in straight patella ligament sutured

Graft passed through the joint

Arthotomy closed

Graft sutured to lateral femoral condyle

Fig. 337(a)   **Fig. 337(b)**   **Fig. 337(c)**

Over the top using the middle third of the straigh patella ligament, the superficial layers of the patella and fascia lata as a graft

The method is ideal for large (over 30 kg weight) and giant breeds of dog. Preparation of the graft is not easy and practice on cadavers is recommended before the actual operation is undertaken. The dog is positioned as in the first 'Over the Top' procedure and the antero–lateral aspect of the stifle is exposed in routine fashion. Two parallel incisions are made in the fascia overlying the patella and these are extended into the bone to a depth of 1 mm using a hacksaw. A sharp chisel is used to skim off the superficial layers of the patella between the 2 incisions, taking care to maintain the ligamentous attachments proximally and distally (Fig. 337a). The 2 parallel incisions are extended distally to free the middle third of the straight patellar ligament as far as its attachment to the tibial crest (Fig. 337a). The incisions are extended proximally and laterally from the patella to produce a strip of fascia lata 1–1.5 cm in diameter and approximately 7 cms in length (Fig. 337a). The strip consisting of fascia lata, superficial layers of the patella and middle third of the straight patella ligament is reflected ventrally. Extreme care must be taken to maintain strong attachment between the patella segment and the proximal and distal ligamentous attachments.

252

The graft is pulled through the defect in the middle of the straight patella ligament (Fig. 337b). The lateral condyle of the femur is exposed and the graft passer positioned as described in the first 'Over the Top' procedure. (Move the graft passer about to make a hole of sufficient size in the caudal joint capsule for the graft to be pulled through). Thread the free end of the graft through the eye of the graft passer and using the instrument, draw the graft through the joint (Fig. 337b). (Because of the patella segment it will not pull through as easily as a fascia lata strip). Pull the graft up tightly and suture the fascia lata to the periosteum of the femoral condyle with monofilament nylon or fine braided wire sutures (Fig. 337c). Excess fascia lata is trimmed off. The defect in the middle third of the straight patellar ligament is closed with one or two simple interrupted sutures and the joint capsule and fascia lata are closed in routine fashion (Fig. 337c).

A Robert Jones bandage is applied for 5 days post operatively. Skin sutures are removed after 10 days and exercise is severely restricted for 6 weeks and then gradually increased. The dog should not be allowed free exercise off a lead for 3 months. Most dogs start to use the affected leg again within 3–4 weeks of surgery and gradually increase the use of the leg, regaining full function within 3–4 months. On follow up of 54 cases treated at this clinic, 35 dogs were sound, 15 had slight or occasional lameness and 4 had persistent lameness. The average follow up period was 2 years with a range from 6 months to 4 years.

Rupture of the collateral ligaments

Collateral ligament injuries are occasionally encountered in the dog and are sometimes associated with rupture of the anterior cruciate ligament.

Manipulation of the joint will reveal abnormal stability in a medial or lateral direction. If the medial collateral ligament has ruptured the tibia may be moved laterally on the femur and the joint may be opened medially (Fig. 338). The converse applies to rupture of the lateral collateral ligament. The joint may be re-stabilized by replacing the collateral

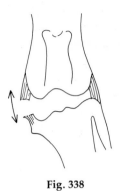

Fig. 338

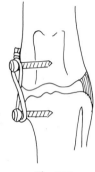

Fig. 339

ligament with a wire prosthesis anchored by a screw placed at the origin and insertion of the ligament (Fig. 339).

Dislocation of the Stifle

Dislocation of the stifle is occasionally encountered. In a series of 5 cases recorded by the author (Denny & Minter 1973), 2 dogs had rupture of both cruciate ligaments and the medial collateral ligament, one had rupture of both cruciate ligaments, another had rupture of both cruciate, collateral ligaments and long digital extensor tendon, and a fifth had rupture of both collateral ligaments. The femur was dislocated caudally on the tibia in those cases with cruciate rupture, and medially or laterally depending on which collateral ligament was ruptured. The joint is stabilized by replacing the anterior cruciate ligament and one of the collateral ligaments. In some cases extra support is given with a plaster cast for 3 weeks.

Luxation of the patella

Luxation of the patella commonly occurs as the result of congenital defects, but it may also be caused by trauma. The luxation may occur medially or laterally, the former being far more common. The cause of medial (congenital) luxation

254

of the patella has not been established, but several workers have shown an association between changes in the hip and stifle deformities (Kodituwakku 1962; Riser *et al* 1969; Putnam 1968). Whatever the primary cause of the condition, a number of deformities exist either alone or in any combination, which result in medial luxation of the patella (Figs. 340, 341). These include coxa vara, lateral bowing of the distal third of the femur, enlarged lateral femoral condyle, shallow or convex femoral trochlea, medial rotation of the tibial tuberosity, and medial bowing of the proximal end of the tibia. If the deformity is minimal, recurrent luxation of the patella occurs but in more severe case it is permanently displaced. The clinical signs of medial luxation (see p. 202) have been described by Lacroix & Riser (1952), Putnam (1968) and Singleton (1969b).

Congenital lateral luxation of the patella also occurs occasionally and again the primary cause has not been ascertained. However, Riser *et al* (1969) described Genu Valgum in giant dogs resulting in lateral luxation of the patella and found that this was due to the lateral metaphyseal portions

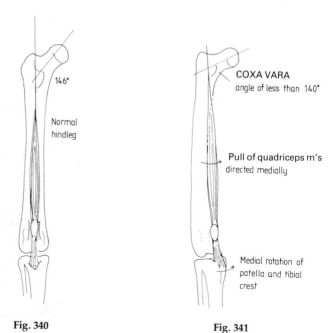

Fig. 340   Fig. 341

of the distal femur and proximal tibia failing to grow as rapidly as their medial counterparts. It was hypothesized that demands for nutrients during growth were greater than the capacity of the vascular system to provide them.

As with medial luxation of the patella deformities exist in the stifle which result in recurrent or permanent lateral luxation. These are basically the converse of those described under medial luxation with the exception that the trochlea is often shallow.

The surgical correction of medial luxation involves the use of one or more techniques to maintain the correct alignment of the patella and its attachments. These techniques include (a) strengthening the stretched or torn lateral joint capsule of the patella by simple suturing (Formston 1932), by construction of a lateral ligament (Jones 1935; Stader 1944; Swain & Miller 1969), by the use of a lateral ligament prosthesis (Leighton 1970), by lateral capsulectomy (Singleton 1957), by capsular overlap (Campbell & Pond 1969) or by fascia lata overlap (Flo & Brinker 1970); (b) tibial tuberosity transplant to correct medial rotation (Singleton, 1957, Mackay & McCune 1967, De Angelis & Hohn 1970), (c) trochlear chondroplasty to deepen the trochlear groove (Singleton 1957; Swain & Miller 1969; De Angelis & Hohn 1970); (d) the use of a prosthesis to increase the height of the medial trochlear ridge (Hickman 1964; Pearson & Ramsay 1963); (e) rotational osteotomy of the tibia and femur (Shuttleworth 1935); (f) medial desmotomy (Lacroix 1930); and (g) patellectomy (Craven 1938; Gibbens 1957).

The same techniques may be employed for lateral luxation but on the medial instead of the lateral aspect of the joint.

In 1973 the author reviewed 91 cases with luxation of the patella. The luxation was medial in 84 cases and lateral in 7. Twelve had traumatic medial luxation. The left leg was affected in 33 cases, the right in 26 and the condition was bilateral in 32. Medial luxation was seen in 22 breeds but the Poodle was most commonly affected. The breed incidence has changed in recent years and it is now the C.K.C. Spaniel that is seen most frequently with this problem, with Yorkshire Terriers, Chihuahua and Papillon taking equal second place. Lateral luxation was seen in 4 breeds: 3 Poodles, 2 Cocker Spaniels, 1 Great Dane and 1 Alsatian. Recently it is the Flat coated Retriever that is affected most often. The overall sex ratio was 54 females to 37 males. Age incidence ranged from 3 months to 12 years, with a peak at 6 months.

Traumatic and recurrent medial luxations of the patella in which there is minimal skeletal deformity are treated by lateral capsular overlap. Permanent medial luxations are corrected by transplanting the tibial crest laterally usually in conjunction with trochlear chondroplasty and medial desmotomy.

Technique for lateral capsular overlap

A lateral parapatellar skin incision is made. The lateral aspect of the joint capsule is incised parallel to the patella and the lateral joint capsule is then overlapped with 2 layers of nylon mattress sutures as shown in Figs 341–343.

Tibial crest transplantation

INDICATIONS

Medial luxation of the patella, Grades 2, 3 and 4 (Singleton, 1969).

Grade 2. Frequent luxation of the patella associated with 15°–30° medial deviation of the tibial crest.

Grade 3. Permanent medial luxation of the patella associated with 30°–60° medial deviation of the tibial crest. The trochlea is usually shallow.

Grade 4. Permanent medial luxation of the patella associated with 60°–90° medial deviation of the tibial crest. The trochlea is absent or convex.

Technique

The dog is placed on its back for surgery. A skin incision is made over the anterolateral aspect of the stifle. The joint capsule is incised lateral to the patella and reflected to allow inspection of the trochlea (Fig. 344). If the trochlea is shallow or absent, it is deepened. The new groove is carved

257

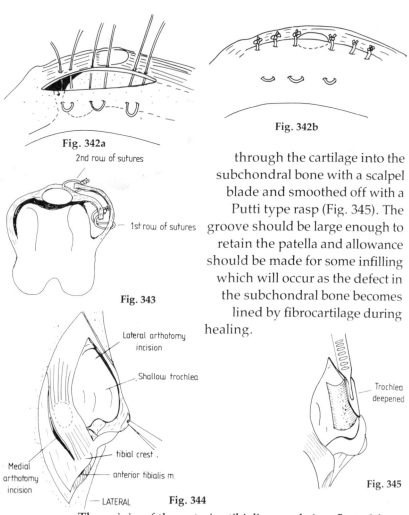

Fig. 342a

2nd row of sutures

1st row of sutures

Fig. 343

Fig. 342b

through the cartilage into the subchondral bone with a scalpel blade and smoothed off with a Putti type rasp (Fig. 345). The groove should be large enough to retain the patella and allowance should be made for some infilling which will occur as the defect in the subchondral bone becomes lined by fibrocartilage during healing.

Lateral arthotomy incision

Shallow trochlea

tibial crest

anterior tibialis m.

Medial arthotomy incision

LATERAL   Fig. 344

Trochlea deepened

Fig. 345

The origin of the anterior tibialis muscle is reflected from the lateral side of the tibial crest. The joint capsule is incised medial to the straight patellar ligament (Fig. 344). The blade of a Liston Bone cutting forceps is slid beneath the straight patellar ligament, the blades are closed on either side of the tibial crest and it is cut free proximally but a periosteal attachment is retained distally (Fig. 346). The crest is levered laterally with a Hohmann retractor to bring it into line with the trochlea and the patella luxation is reduced (Fig. 347a).

A tunnel is drilled through the tibial crest and proximal tibia from lateral to medial, using a straight traumatic needle as a drill bit. A length of 24 or 20 gauge wire is passed

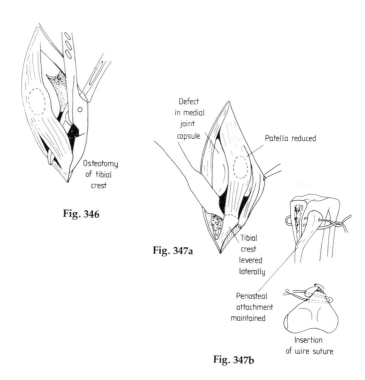

Fig. 346

Osteotomy of tibial crest

Defect in medial joint capsule

Patella reduced

Fig. 347a

Tibial crest levered laterally

Periosteal attachment maintained

Insertion of wire suture

Fig. 347b

through the tunnel. A second tunnel is drilled from the medial side of the proximal tibia, this does not penetrate the tibial crest but merges just caudal to it (Fig. 347b). The medial end of the wire is passed back through this tunnel and the free ends of the wire are twisted tight drawing the tibial crest down firmly in its new lateral position. The medial and lateral arthrotomy incisions are closed next. Excess joint capsule on the lateral side of the patella is overlapped with a double row of sutures while the defect in the medial joint capsule (Fig. 347) is covered with a layer of subcutaneous fascia. The anterior tibialis muscle is secured to the straight patella ligament or adjacent joint capsule with mattress sutures. The subcutaneous tissues and skin are closed in routine fashion.

POST OPERATIVE CARE

A support bandage is applied for a week post operatively. Antibiotic cover is given for 5 days and skin sutures are removed at 10 days. Exercise is restricted for 4 weeks and

259

then gradually increased. In dogs with bilateral patella luxation, an interval of 2 months is left between operations on each stifle.

Complications
1   Re–luxation of the patella may result from:
(a) Failure to transplant the tibial crest in normal alignment with the trochlea.
(b) Failure to adequately immobilise the tibial crest in its new position.
(c) Failure to provide a trochlea of sufficient depth.
2   Inability to fully extend the stifle joint. This complication is generally seen in dogs with Grade IV medial luxation when surgical correction has been attempted towards the end of growth or after 1 year of age. Ideally, surgical correction should be undertaken at 4–5 months of age, before contracture of the caudal muscles of the stifle has resulted in permanent joint deformity with inability to extend the stifle.

Genu valgum in giant dogs resulting in lateral luxation of the patella may be corrected by placing a stable or compression wire across the medial aspect of the distal femoral epiphyseal plate. The implant is removed as soon as the deformity has been corrected usually between 4 and 8 weeks.

Osteochondritis dissecans (OCD) of the stifle joint (Denny and Gibbs 1980)

Osteochondritis Dissecans (OCD) is a fairly uncommon cause of stifle lameness. The OCD lesion is found in either the medial or lateral condyle of the femur. The breed incidence is listed in order of decreasing frequency.

Breed incidence
Wolfhound
Labrador
Staff Bull Terrier
Alsatian
Greyhound
Retriever

260

Standard Poodle

Chow

Male dogs are more frequently affected than females. There is a gradual onset of lameness at approximately 5 months of age.

Animals with bilateral lesions have a crouching action and difficulty in rising. There is discomfort and crepitus on manipulation of the stifle but *no* instability.

In the radiographic diagnosis, the AP view is most useful to demonstrate an erosion in the femoral condyle.

On the lateral view, look for calcified fragments within the joint.

Surgical treatment is recommended in most cases, however, OCD of the stifle like the shoulder does not cause the rapid and severe osteoarthrosis that is encountered when the elbow or hock are affected.

Arthrodesis of the stifle

Arthrodesis of the stifle is occasionally indicated for the relief of painful osteoarthritis caused by joint infection.

The anterior aspect of the joint is exposed and the patella removed. The articular surfaces of the femur and tibia are removed together with the menisci. A cancellous bone graft is packed in the joint space and a plate applied to the anterior aspect of the femur and tibia. The stifle is fixed in a slightly flexed position (Fig. 348).

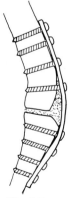

Fig. 348

Dogs accommodate to the arthrodesis well although there may be a tendency to knuckle at the digits for the first three to four weeks.

Fractures of the tibia

Fractures of the proximal tibia are described under surgery of the stifle joint while those involving the distal tibia are described under Surgery of the Hock.

Mid-shaft fractures are usually oblique or spiral and the fibula is invariably fractured also. As there is little soft tissue cover on the medial aspect of the tibia the fractures are often compound.

Stable fractures can be treated by external support in a plaster cast, however the majority require open reduction and internal fixation using a plate. An anteromedial skin incision is made and the skin flap reflected to expose the medial aspect of the tibia. The plate must be carefully contoured to the shape of the tibia otherwise lateral deviation of the foot will occur (Fig. 349).

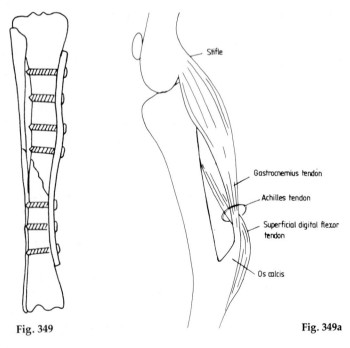

Stifle

Gastrocnemius tendon

Achilles tendon

Superficial digital flexor tendon

Os calcis

Fig. 349   Fig. 349a

ACHILLES TENDON INJURY

The Achilles tendon consists of the tendons of the gastrocnemius muscle and the superficial digital flexor muscle (Fig. 349a). The gastrocnemius tendon inserts on the tuber calcis while the superficial digital flexor tendon curves over the tip of the os calcis as a broad flat band. A bursa lies between the tendon and the tip of the os calcis.

Displacement of the tendon of the superficial digital flexor muscle (Bernard 1977, Bennett & Campbell 1979 and Vaughan 1979).

Displacement of the tendon of the superficial digital flexor occurs spontaneously or through direct trauma. Rupture of the medial retinaculum allows the tendon to displace in a lateral direction in most cases. There is a sudden onset of lameness, swelling and pain over the point of the hock and the tendon can be easily returned to its normal position. In untreated cases, extensive fibrosis and tenosynovitis occur.

A curved incision is made over the medial side of the os calcis, the tendon is reduced and the torn retinacular attachments repaired with single interrupted sutures of fine monofilament nylon. In chronic cases, the stretched and fibrosed medial retinaculum is incised parallel with the tendon and overlapped with two layers of sutures in a similar way to the capsular overlap procedure described on page 258 for patellar luxation. Post-operatively, the hock is immobilized with a Robert Jones bandage for 2 weeks and exercise should be restricted for 4 weeks.

Rupture of the achilles tendon (Bloomberg, Hough and Howard 1976; Vaughan 1979)

Rupture of the Achilles tendon usually occurs through direct trauma, the dog striking its leg on a piece of sharp metal for example. Often there is a small skin wound just proximal to the os calcis. However, rupture of the tendon produces an obvious postural deformity; the hock is 'dropped' and a plantigrade stance occurs if the dog attempts to bear weight on the leg. The hock can be hyper-flexed and the Achilles tendon remains flaccid instead of becoming taut. Often the cut ends of the tendon can be palpated subcutaneously some distance from the original site of injury.

SURGICAL REPAIR OF THE ACHILLES TENDON

Before suturing the tendon, the hock should be fixed in extension; this facilitates the repair and avoids undue tension on the sutures during the healing process. A skin incision is made over the lateral aspect of the Achilles tendon and extended down over the os calcis. An incision is made in the lateral retinaculum of the superficial digital flexor tendon to allow medial displacement of the tendon and exposure of the caudal surface of the os calcis. The hock is fully extended and a screw is driven through the os calcis into the distal tibia (Fig. 349b). The lag screw principle is

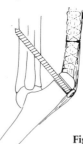

Fig. 349b

used, the hole in the os calcis being overdrilled so that the screw thread grips in the tibia only. It is important to retract and protect the soft tissues between the os calcis and caudal tibia during preparation of the screw hole and insertion of the screw. The severed ends of the gastrocnemius and superficial digital flexor tendons are identified and each tendon is repaired separately using monofilament nylon. Two types of tendon suture patterns are commonly used—Bunnells' pattern described in 1940 has stood the test of time (see Fig. 349d) while the locking loop tendon/ligament suture (Fig. 349e,f) (Pennington 1979) is easier to apply and allows more accurate apposition of the tendon ends.

The lateral attachments of the superficial digital flexor tendon to the os calcis are repaired with interrupted sutures

264

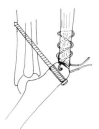

Fig. 349c

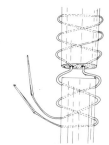

Fig. 349d

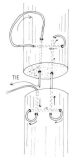

TIE

Fig. 349e

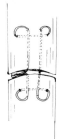

Fig. 349f

of monofilament nylon. The rest of the wound closure is routine. A Robert Jones bandage is then applied for 10 days post–operatively. Exercise is restricted until the lag screw is removed at 4 weeks and is then gradually increased.

MANAGEMENT OF LONGSTANDING ACHILLES TENDON RUPTURE

The principles of treatment are the same as for recent injuries. However contracture of the tendons will have occurred which often prevents complete apposition of the ends. A defect should be bridged with carbon fibre (Johnson & Johnson) which acts as a scaffold and induces collagen formation across the defect (Jenkins *et al* 1977).

AVULSION OF THE TENDON OF INSERTION OF THE GASTROCNEMIUS MUSCLE

The presenting signs are the same as for rupture of the Achilles tendon but there is no wound, just a swelling over the os calcis. A radiograph may show that the tendon has been avulsed with a small fragment of bone. The hock is fixed in extension with a lag screw as described under Achilles tendon rapture. A Bunnell suture of monofilament wire is inserted into the gastrocnemius tendon, the ends of the wire are passed through a transverse drill hole in the os calcis and then tightened (Fig. 349c).

SURGERY OF THE HOCK

The hock is a composite joint consisting of 7 tarsal bones and their related soft tissues. The tarsal bones are arranged in three irregular rows (Figs 350–351). The tibio-tarsal articulation is ginglymus and it is here that most motion occurs. The intertarsal and tarso-metatarsal articulations are arthrodia and normally movement between them is minimal.

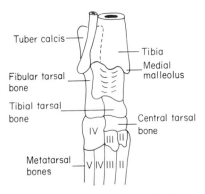

Fig. 350. Cranial view right hock

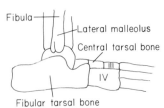

Fig. 351. Lateral view right hock

The clinical signs of injuries to the canine hock are well recognized, particularly in the racing Greyhound. Injury to the hock may result in:

1 *Fractures*
(a) Fracture of the distal epiphysis of the tibia.
(b) Malleolar fractures.
(c) Fracture of the tuber calcis of the fibular tarsal bone.
(d) Fracture of the central tarsal bone.
(e) Occasional fractures of the other tarsal bones.

266

2   *Dislocations and subluxations*

(a) Tibiotarsal dislocation, often associated with a malleolar fracture.

(b) Intertarsal subluxation.

(c) Tarso-metatarsal subluxation or dislocation.

1(a) Fracture of the distal epiphysis of the tibia.

Closed reduction and external fixation of this fracture is difficult owing to the small size of the distal fragment. The fracture is therefore usually treated by open reduction. A medial or lateral approach is used depending on the direction of displacement of the fragments. Fixation may be obtained in the following ways:

(i) Crossed Kirschner wires. These wires are inserted up through the malleoli (Fig. 352). Rush pins may be used in a similar way in larger dogs. Usually further external support is necessary until the fracture has healed.

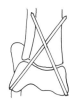 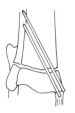 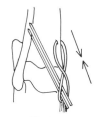

| Fig. 352 | Fig. 353 | Fig. 354 |

(ii) The wire tension band (Muller *et al* 1970) has been used by the author for treatment of this fracture. Following reduction, two Kirschner wires are inserted up through the medial malleolus (Fig. 353); these provide axial stability. A hole is drilled through the tibia proximal to the fracture line, a length of stainless steel wire is passed through the proximal end of the medial collateral ligament, the ends are brought across the medial side of the fracture in a figure of 8 fashion before being passed through the hole in the tibia. The ends of the wire are tightened thus compressing the fracture (Figs 353–354).

This method gives stable internal fixation and post-operatively no external support is necessary.

1(b) Malleolar fractures

Fracture of a malleolus is often associated with dislocation or subluxation of the tibio-tarsal joint. The malleolus is the point of origin of the collateral ligament and this ligament causes distraction of the fragments. The fracture is therefore treated by open reduction and internal fixation using either a screw (Fig. 355) (Leighton 1957; Holt 1976), rush pin (Lawson 1958) or wire tension band.

Fig. 355

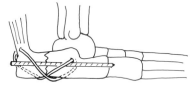

Fig. 356

1(c) Fracture of the tuber calcis of the fibular tarsal bone

The pull of the gastrocnemius muscle results in marked distraction of the fragments. The fracture is treated by open reduction using a caudo-lateral approach.

Fixation is achieved using a Steinman pin or Kirschner wires in combination with a tension band wire (Fig. 356).

1(d) Fracture of the central tarsal bone

The treatment of fractures of the central tarsal bone was described by Bateman in 1958.

In a more recent publication, Dee *et al* (1978), a classification of fractures of the central tarsal bone was presented together with treatment and prognosis. The fractures were grouped into 5 types:

Type 1 An anterior slab fracture with no displacement is treated by external fixation.

Type 2 An anterior slab fracture with anterior and proximal displacement is treated by open reduction and fixation with a single lag screw (Figs 357, 358)

Type 3 A fracture in the saggital plane with or without anterior displacement of the medial fragment is treated by open reduction and fixation with a single lag screw.

Type 4 This fracture is a combination of Types 2 and 3, in which there is anterior displacement of a slab, in conjunction with a larger medially displaced fragment. The fracture is treated by open reduction and fixation with two lag screws.

Type 5 The central tarsal bone is severely comminuted and displaced. Treatment is by closed reduction and external support.

The prognosis for Types 1 and 2 fractures is good, for Types 3 and 4, fair to good and Type 5, poor. External support is provided in all cases treated by internal fixation.

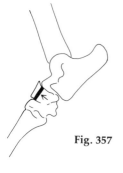

Fig. 357

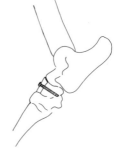

Fig. 358

2(a) Tibiotarsal dislocation

Treatment of this injury when associated with fracture of a malleolus has already been described.

The tibia most commonly luxates medially due to rupture of the lateral collateral ligament (Fig. 359a). Closed reduction and immobilization in a plaster cast may be carried out. However, if the joint is unstable or irreducible, following open reduction it may be stabilized by replacing the collateral ligament with a wire prosthesis. A screw is placed at the origin and insertion of the collateral ligament and a wire figure of 8 suture placed around them (Fig. 359b).

Dislocation of the hock may occur as a complication of severe abrasive injury. For example, the dog which has been dragged along the road by a car, the soft tissues of the lateral hock and foot and varying degrees of bone are planed

269

away as a result (Fig. 360). Initial debridement is carried out and the foot protected with a Robert Jones bandage. The bandage is changed once every 2 or 3 days. Once discharge has ceased and the wound is beginning to fill with healthy granulation tissue, a cast is applied from the toes to just below the stifle. It is suprising how well some of these wounds heal just with the protection afforded by the cast. If hock instability persists, then replacement of the collateral ligament can be carried out using screws and a figure of 8 wire but this should not be done until the wound has almost healed.

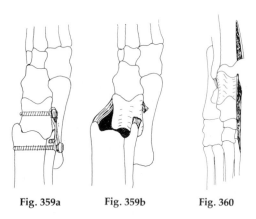

Fig. 359a   Fig. 359b   Fig. 360

2(b and c) Intertarsal and tarso metatarsal subluxation

Damage to the plantar ligaments of the hock may result in intertarsal subluxation (Fig. 361) or tarso-metatarsal subluxation (Lawson 1960; Arwedsson 1954; Campbell *et al* 1976). Treatment usually involves arthodesis of the affected joints. Achieve a bloodless field for surgery (see OCD of the hock). The joints are exposed by a caudolateral skin incision and the articular cartilage removed. Following reduction, a variety of methods of fixation may be employed (Arwedsson 1954). An olecranon screw has been used for intertarsal subluxation (Fig. 362) (Lawson 1960). Alternatively, a plate may be applied to the lateral aspect of the joint, or a Steinman pin and wire tension band may be used for fixation (Fig. 363). The wire is passed transversely through the caudal aspect of the fibular tarsal bone and the

270

4th tarsal bone. Alternatively, the distal end of the tension band wire can be anchored in the head of the lateral metatarsal bone.

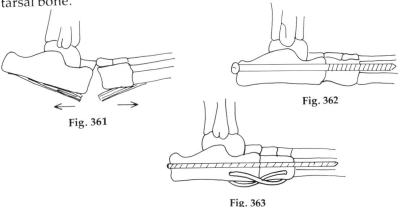

Fig. 361

Fig. 362

Fig. 363

Osteochondritis dissecans of the hock joint (Olsson 1975; Mason & Lavelle 1979; Denny 1981.)

Osteochondritis dissecans of the hock joint has been recognised as a cause of lameness with increasing frequency during the past few years. The onset is between 4 and 10 months of age. The lesion is located in the articular surface of the medial ridge of the tibial tarsal bone (Fig. 364) and the condition is often bilateral. Occasionally, however, the lateral ridge of the tibial tarsal bone is affected (Mason 1978). The condition is seen most frequently in Labradors, Retrievers, Rottweilers and Irish Wolfhounds.

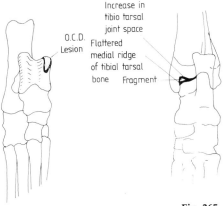

O.C.D. Lesion

Increase in tibio tarsal joint space
Flattered medial ridge of tibial tarsal bone   Fragment

Fig. 364

Fig. 365

malleolar fractures or injuries to the collateral ligaments. The operation is also used in the relief of pain caused by advanced osterarthritis.

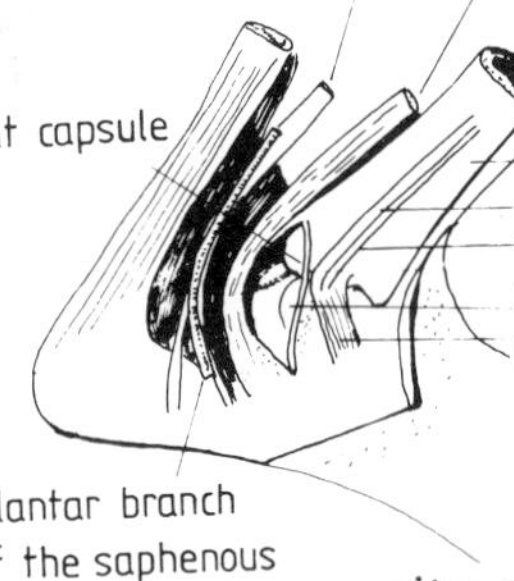

The tibial tarsal joint is exposed by a medial or lateral incision and the articular surfaces removed. A separate small incision is made on the caudal aspect of the tibial tarsal bone and the hock positioned for fusion at 135°–145°. A hole is drilled up through the tibial tarsal bone into the medullary cavity of the tibia. This is tapped to allow insertion of a cancellous screw for fixation (Fig. 368). A tension band of 20-gauge wire is then placed from the tuber calcis to the distal tibia to help relieve excessive stress on the screw. External support is given with a plaster cast for four weeks following surgery.

Labels on figure:
Tibial nerve
Flexor hallucis longus tendon
Joint capsule
Tibia
Flexor digitorum longus
Tibialis caudalis tendon
Tibiotarsal bone
Medial collateral ligament
Plantar branch of the saphenous artery and vein

Amputation of the hind leg

The indications for amputation of a limb have already been described on page 192. Amputation of the hind limb is performed through the proximal third of the femur. A semi-circular skin incision is made on the lateral aspect of the leg extending from the distal third of the thigh to the stifle joint. The leg is lifted by an assistant and a similar skin incision is made on the medial aspect of the thigh. The medial skin flap is reflected and the femoral artery and vein identified just cranial to the pectineus muscle. Both vessels are ligated. Early ligation of these vessels reduces haemorrhage during the subsequent amputation. The limb is then lowered. The biceps femoris, semi-membranosus and semitendinosus muscles are sectioned just proximal to the stifle together with the sciatic nerve and and distal femoral artery. The sartorius muscle and quadriceps are sectioned to complete exposure of the distal femur. The muscle bellies are bluntly reflected from the femur with a swab and exposure of the proximal shaft completed by elevation of the adductor

274

muscle. The amputation is completed by section of the femur through the proximal third of the shaft with a saw. Wound closure is as described under Amputation of the forelimb.

REFERENCES

ARNOCZKY S.P., TARVIN G.B., MARSHALL J.L. & SALTZMAN B. (1979) The Over-the-Top Procedure: a technique for anterior cruciate ligament substitution in the dog. *J. Am. Anim. Hosp. Ass.* **15,** 283.

ARWEDSSON, G. (1954) *J. Amer. vet. med. Ass.* **124,** 21.

BARDENS J. & HARDWICK H. (1968) New observations on the diagnosis and causes of hip dysplasia. *Vet. Med./Small Anim. Clin.* **63,** 238.

BATEMAN J.K. (1958) *Vet. Rec.* **70,** 621.

BATEMAN J.K. (1960) *Vet Rec.* **72,** 893.

BATEMAN J.K. (1964) *Vet. Rec.* **76,** 201.

BENNETT D. & CAMPBELL J.R. (1979) Unusual soft tissue orthopaedic problems in the dog. *J. small Anim. Pract.* **20,** 27.

BERNARD M.A. (1977) Superficial digital flexor tendon injury in the dog. *Can. vet. J.* **18,** 105.

BETTS C.W. & WALKER M. (1975) *J. small Anim. Pract.* **16,** 21.

BLOOMBERG M.S., HOUGH J.D. & HOWARD D.R. (1976) Repair of a severed Achilles tendon in a dog: a case report. *J. Am. Anim. Hosp. Ass.* **12,** 841.

BOWEN J.M., LEWIS R.E., KNELLER S.K., WILSON R.C. & ARNOLD R.A. (1972) *J. Am. Vet. Med. Ass.* **161,** 899.

BRINKER W.O. (1965) *Canine Surgery,* First Archibald Edition. American Veterinary Medical Publications Inc, Santa Barbara, California.

BRINKER W.O. (1971) Corrective osteotomy procedures for treatment of canine hip dysplasia. *Vet. Clinics of N. America,* **1,** 467.

BRINKER W.O. (1975) in *Current Techniques in Small Animal Surgery,* ed. BJORAB M.J. Lea & Febiger, Philadelphia.

BROOK G.B. (1932) *Vet. Rec.* **12,** 240.

BROWN G.S. & BIGGART J.F. (1975) Plate fixation of iliac shaft fractures in the dog. *J. Am. Vet. Med. Ass.* **167,** 472.

BUNNELL S. (1940) Primary repair of severed tendons. *Am. J. Surg.* **47,** 502.

CAMPBELL J.R. (1977) Femorotibial surgery in the dog. *Vet. Rec.* **101,** 318.

CAMPBELL J.R., BENNETT D. & LEE R. (1976) *J. small Anim. Pract.* **17,** 427.

CAMPBELL J.R. & POND M.J. (1969) *J. small Anim. Pract.* **10,** 320.

CARLIN I. (1926) *Arch. wiss. prakt. Tierbalk.* **54,** 420.

CRAVEN N.S. (1938) *N. Am. Vet.* **19,** 55.

DAVIS P.E. (1967) *Aust. Vet. J.* **43,** 519.

DE ANGELIS M. & HOHN R.B. (1970) *J. Am. Vet. Med. Ass.* **156,** 587.

DEE J.F., DEE J. & PIERMATTEI D.C. (1976) *J. Amer. Anim. Hosp. Ass.* **12,** 398.

DENNY H.R. (1971) *J. small Anim. Pract.* **12,** 613.

DENNY H.R. (1975) *J. small Anim. Pract.* **16,** 173.

DENNY H.R. (1976) Surgery of the canine hip. *The Veterinary Annual,* 17th edn, p. 156. Wright Scientechnic, Bristol.

DENNY H.R. (1978) Pelvic fractures in the dog: a review of 123 cases. *J. small Anim. Pract.* **19,** 151.

DENNY H.R. (1981) Osteochondritis dissecans of the hock joint in the dog. The Veterinary Annual, 21st Ed. Wright Scientechnica, Bristol. p. 224.

DENNY H.R. & GIBBS C. (1980) Osteochondritis dissecans of the canine stifle joint. *J. small Anim. Pract.* **22**, 317.

DENNY H.R. & GOODSHIP A.E. (1980) Replacement of the anterior cruciate ligament with carbon fibre in the dog. *J. small Anim. Pract.* **21**, 279.

DENNY H.R. & MINTER H.M. (1973) Recurrent coxofemoral luxation in the dog. *The Veterinary Annual,* 14th edn, p. 220. Wright Scientechnic, Bristol.

DENNY H.R. & MINTER H.M. (1973) The long term results of surgery of canine stifle disorders. *J. small Anim. Pract.* **14**, 695–713.

DINGWALL J.S. & SUMNER-SMITH G. (1971) *J. small Anim. Pract.* **12**, 665.

DUFF R. & CAMPBELL H.M. (1977) Long-term results of excision arthroplasty of the canine hip. *Vet. Rec.* **101**, 181.

EMERY M.A. & ROSTRUP D. (1960) *Can. J. Surg.* **4**, 111.

FLO G.F. & BRINKER W.O. (1970) *J. Am. Vet. Med. Ass.* **156**, 595.

FORMSTON C. (1932) *Vet. Rec.* **12**, 410.

GIBBENS R. (1957) *J. Am. Vet. Med. Ass.* **131**, 557.

GRONDALEN J. (1969) Fractura pelvis hos hund. *Nord Vet. Med.* **21**, 505.

GUPTA B.V. & BRINKER W.O. (1969) *J. Am. Vet. Med. Ass.* **154**, 1057.

HAUPTMAN J., HULSE D. & CHITWOOD J. (1976) Indications for stabilization of sacroiliac luxations in the dog and cat. *Vet. Med./Small animal Clin.* **00**, 1415.

HEFFRON L.E. (1976) A study of certain aspects of rupture of the canine anterior cruciate ligament. MVM Thesis, University of Glasgow.

HENRICSON B., LJUNGGREN G. & OLSSON S.A. (1972) Canine hip dysplasia in Sweden. Incidence and genetics. *Acta Radiol. Suppl.* **175**, 317.

HENRY J.D. (1975) A modified technique for pectineal tenotomy in the dog. *J. Am. Vet. Med. Ass.* **163**, 465.

HENRY W.B. & WADSWORTH P. (1975) Pelvic osteotomy in the treatment of subluxation associated with hip dysplasia. *J. Am. Anim. Hosp. Ass.* **11**, 636.

HICKMAN J. (1964) *Veterinary Orthopaedics.* Oliver & Boyd, London.

HICKMAN J. (1975) *J. small Anim. Pract.* **16**, 455.

HINKO P.J. (1974) *J. Am. Anim. Hosp. Ass.* **10**, 61.

HOHN R.B. & MILLER J.M. (1967) *J. Am. Vet. Med. Ass.* **150**, 1133.

HOHN R.B. & NEWTON C. (1972) Personal communication.

HOLT P.E. (1976) *Vet. Rec.* **99**, 335.

HULSE D.A., WILSON J.W. & BUTLER H.C. (1974) *J. Am. Anim. Hosp. Ass.* **10**, 29.

JENKINS D.H.R., FORSTER I.W., McKIBBIN B. & RALIS Z.A. (1977) Induction of tendon and ligament formation by carbon implants. *J. Bone Jt. Surg.* **59B**, 53.

JOHNSON F.L. (1960) *J. Am. Vet. Med. Ass.* **137**, 646.

JONES V.B. (1935) *Vet. J.* **91**, 281.

KIRKBRIDE L.M. & CARTER J.G. (1970) Fracture of the inominate bone in a male mongrel dog. *Vet. Rec.* **87**, 643.

KNECHT C.D. (1976) Evolution of surgical techniques for cruciate ligament rupture in animals. *J. Am. Anim. Hosp. Ass.* **12**, 717.

KNIGHT G.L. (1956) *Vet. Rec.* **68**, 415.

KNOWLES A.T., KNOWLES J.O. & KNOWLES R.P. (1953) *J. Am. Vet. Med. Ass.* **123**, 508.

KODITUWAKKU G.E. (1962) *Vet. Rec.* **74**, 1499.

LACROIX V.J. (1930) *N. Am. Vet.* **11**, 47.

LACROIX V.J. & RISER L.H. (1952) *Canine Surgery,* 3rd edn. American Veterinary Publications Inc. Illinois, USA.

LAWSON D.D. (1958) *Vet. Rec.* **70**, 763.

LAWSON D.D. (1960) *J. small Anim. Pract.* **1**, 179.

LAWSON D.D. (1963) The radiographic diagnosis of hip dysplasia in the dog. *Vet. Rec.* **75**, 445.

LAWSON D.D. (1965) *J. small Anim. Pract.* **6**, 57.

LEE R. (1970) A study of the radiographic and histological changes occuring in Legg-Calve-Perthes disease in the dog. *J. small Anim. Pract.* **11**, 621.

LEE R. & FRY P.D. (1969) Some observations on the occurrence of Legge-Calve-Perthes disease (coxoplana) in the dog, and an evaluation of excision arthroplasty as a method of treatment. *J. small Anim. Pract.* **10**, 309.

LEIGHTON R.C. (1957) *Cornell Vet.* **47**, 396.

LEIGHTON R.L. (1968) The surgical treatment of some pelvic fractures. *J. Am. Vet. Med. Ass.* **153**, 1739.

LEIGHTON R.L. (1970) *Vet. Med.* **65**, 365.

LEONARD E.P. (1971) *Orthopaedic Surgery of the Dog and Cat,* 2nd edn. W.B. Saunders Company, Philadelphia.

LEWIS D.G. (1974) A modified tendon transfer technique for stabilising the canine stifle joint after rupture of the cruciate ligament(s). *Vet. Rec.* **94**, 3.

LJUNGGREN G. (1966) A comparative study of conservative and surgical treatment of Legg-Perthe's disease in the dog. *J. Am. Anim. Hosp. Ass.* **2**, 6.

LJUNGGREN G. (1967) Legge-Perthe's disease. *Acta Orthop. Scand. Suppl.* **95**, 1967.

LUST G., CRAIG P.H., ROSS G.E. & GEARY J.C. (1972) *Cornell Vet.* **62**, 628.

MACKAY N.W. & McCUNE R.F. (1967) *Mod. vet. Pract.* **48**, 52.

MASON T.A. & LAVELLE R.B. (1979) *J. small anim. Pract.* **20**, 423.

MORRIS R.E. (1970) Surgical repair of the pelvis in a dog. *Vet. Rec.* **86**, 559.

MULLER M.E., ALLGOWER M. & WILLENEGGER H. (1970) *Manual of Internal Fixation.* Springer-Verlag, Berlin Heidelberg New York.

NISSEN K.I. (1971) The rationale of early osteotomy for idiopathic cox-arthrosis (epichondro-osteoarthrosis of the hip). *Clinical Orthopaedics,* **77**, 98.

OLMSTEAD M.L., HOHN R.B., TURNER T.T. (1981) Technique for total hip replacement. *Vet. Surg.* **10**, 44.

OLSSON S.E. (1975) Lameness in the dog. *Proceedings Am. Anim. Hosp. Ass.* **42**, 363.

ORMROD A.N. (1963) *Vet. Rec.* **75**, 375.

PAATSAMA S. (1952) Ligament injuries inthe canine stifle joint. Dissertation, University of Helsinki.

PAATSAMA S., RISSANEN P. & ROKKANEN P. (1967) Legge-Perthe's disease in the dog. *J. Small Animal Practice.* **8**, 215.

PAATSAMA S., RISSANEN P. & ROKKANEN P. (1969) Microangiographic changes in Legg-Perthe's disease in young dogs. *Scand. J. Clin. Lab. Invest.* **23**, Suppl. 108, 95.

PEARSON P.T. & RAMSEY F.K. (1963) *J. Am. Vet. Med. Ass.* **143**, 843.

PENNINGTON D.G. (1979) The locking loop tendon suture. *Plas. & Reconstr. Surg.* **63**, 648.

PETIT G.D. & SLATTER D.H. (1973) *J. Am. Vet. Med. Ass.* **163**, 242.

PIDDUCK H. & WEBBON P.M. (1978) The genetic control of Perthes disease in Toy Poodles—a working hypothesis. *J. small Anim. Pract.* **19**, 729–733.

PIERMATTEI D.C. & GREELEY R.G. (1966) *An Atlas of Surgical Approaches to the Bones of the Dog and Cat.* W.B. Saunders Company, Philadelphia.

POND M.J. (1973) *J. small Anim. Pract.* **14**, 795.

POND M.J. (1975) in *Current Techniques in Small Animal Surgery*, ed. BOJRAB M.J. Lea & Febiger, Philadelphia.

POND M.J. & CAMPBELL J.R. (1972) *J. small Anim. Pract.* **13**, 1.

PUTNAM G. (1968) MSc Thesis, University of Guelph.

RATHOS S.S. (1960) *Mich. St. Univ. Vet.* **20**, 128.

RISER W.H. (1963) Necrosis of the femoral head. *J. Am. Vet. Med. Ass.* **142**, 1024.

RISER W.H. (1973) The dysplastic hip joint, its radiographic and histologic development. *J. Am. Vet. Radiol.* **14**, 35.

RISER W.H., PARKES L.J., RHODES W.H. & SHIRER J.F. (1969) *J. Am. Vet. Radiol. Soc.* **10**, 28.

ROBINS G.M. (1970) *J. small anim. Pract.* **11**, 813.

ROBINS G.M., DINGWALL J.S. & SIMNER-SMITH G. (1973) The plating of pelvic fractures in the dog. *Vet. Rec.* **93**, 550.

ROBINS G.M. (1978) *Aust. Vet. J.* **54**, 272.

SANDERS N. (1962) *Aust Vet. J.* **38**, 239.

SHUTTLEWORTH A.C. (1935) *Vet. Rec.* **47**, 765.

SINGLETON W.B. (1957) *Vet. Rec.* **69**, 1387.

SINGLETON W.B. (1963) *Can. vet. J.* **4**, 142.

SINGLETON W.B. (1969a) *J. small Anim. Pract.* **10**, 269.

SINGLETON W.B. (1969b) *J. small Anim. Pract.* **10**, 59.

SMITH K.W. (1971) Legg-Perthe's disease. *Vet. Clinics N. America,* **1**, 479.

SPRUELL J.S.A. (1961) Excision arthroplasty as a method of treatment of hip joint diseases in the dog. *Vet. Rec.* **13**, 573.

STADER O. (1944) *N. Am. Vet.* **25**, 757.

STOLL G.S., SINIBALDI K.R., DE ANGELIS M.P. & ROSEN H. (1975) A technique for tibiotarsal arthrodesis in utilizing cancellous bone screws in small animals. *J. Am. An. Hosp. Ass.* **11**, 185.

STRANDE A. (1966) *J. small Anim. Pract.* **7**, 351.

SUMNER-SMITH G. & DINGWALL J.G. (1973) *J. Am. An. Hosp. Ass.* **9**, 171.

SWAIN S.F. & MILLER L.N. (1969) *Vet. Med.* **64**, 512.

VAN OOSTEROM R.A.A. (1982) Intra-articular Graft Passer. *Vet. Surg.* **11**, 132.

VAUGHAN L.C. (1963) *Vet. Rec.* **75**, 537.

VAUGHAN L.C. (1969) *J. small Anim. Pract.* **10**, 363.

VAUGHAN L.C. (1979) Muscle and tendon injuries in dogs. *J. small Anim. Pract.* **20**, 711.

VAUGHAN L.C. & BOWDEN N.L.R. (1964) *J. small Anim. Pract.* **5**, 167

VAUGHAN L.C. & FORMSTON C. (1975) *J. small Anim. Pract.* **14**, 267.

VAUGHAN L.C., CLAYTON JONES D.G. & LANE J.G. (1975) Pectineus muscle resection as a treatment for hip dysplasia in dogs. *Vet. Rec.* **96**, 145.

WALLACE L.J. (1971) Pectineus tendonectomy or tenotomy for treating canine hip dysplasia. *Vet. Clinics N. America,* **1**, 455.

WHEATON L.G., HOHN R.B. & HARRISON J.W. (1973) The surgical treatment of acetabular fractures in the dog. *J. Am. Vet. Med. Ass.* **162,** 385.

WHITICK W.G. (1974) *Canine Orthopaedics.* Lea & Febiger, Philadelphia.

WITHROW S., DE ANGELIS M., ARNOCZKY S. & ROSEN H. (1976) *J. Am. Vet. Med. Ass.* **168,** 132.

ZAKIEWICZ M. (1967) *Vet. Rec.* **81,** 538.

Index